S0-BNR-024

EXERCISE ACTIVITIES for the ELDERLY

Kay Flatten, P.E.D.
Barbara Wilhite, Ed.D.
Eleanor Reyes-Watson, M.A.

Illustrated by Rini Twait

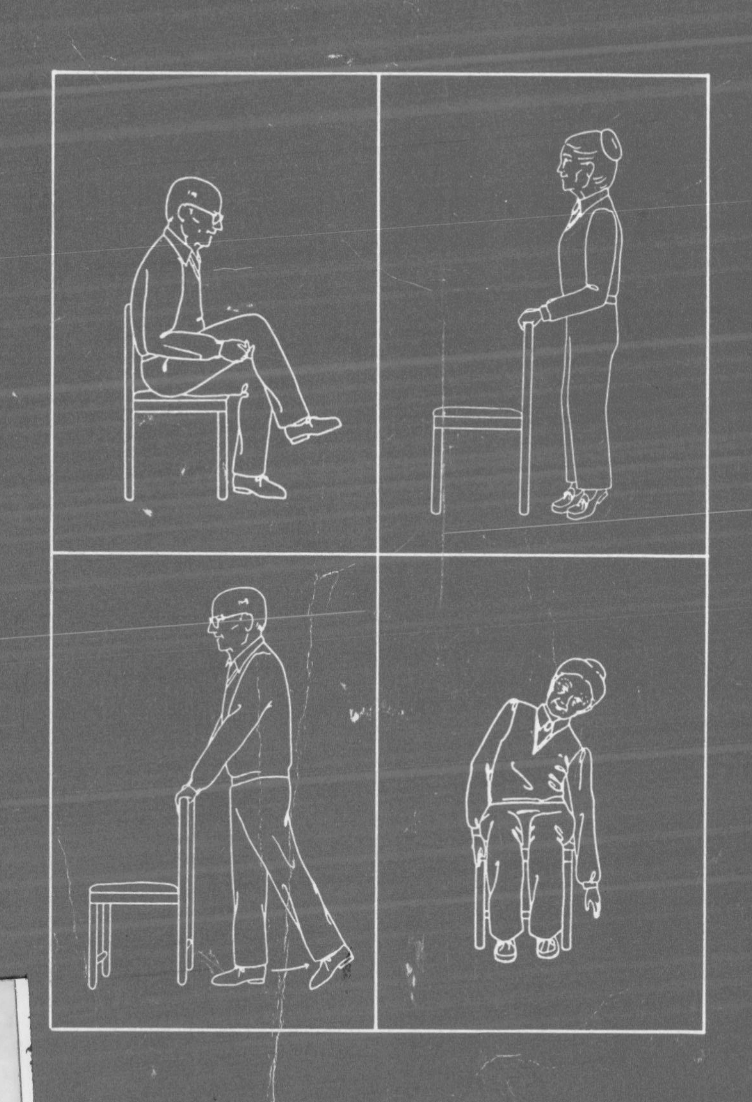

[Sp]ringer Series on Adulthood and Aging

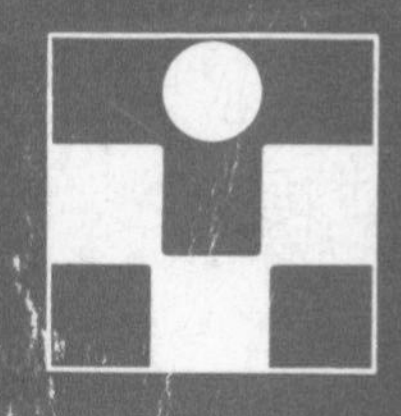

Springer Series on ADULTHOOD and AGING

Vol. 1 **Adult Day Care** *Philip G. Weiler et al. O.P.*

Vol. 2 **Counseling Elders and Their Families:** Practical Techniques for Applied Gerontology *John J. Herr and John H. Weakland*

Vol. 3 **Becoming Old:** An Introduction to Social Gerontology *John C. Morgan*

Vol. 4 **The Projective Assessment of Aging Method (PAAM)** *Bernard D. Starr, Marcella Bakur Weiner, and Marilyn Rabetz*

Vol. 5 **Ethnicity and Aging** *Donald E. Gelfand and Alfred J. Kutzik, with 25 contributors*

Vol. 6 **Gerontology Instruction in Higher Education** *David A. Peterson and Christopher R. Bolton O.P.*

Vol. 7 **Nontraditional Therapy and Counseling with the Aging** *S. Stansfeld Sargent et al.*

Vol. 8 **The Aging Network:** Programs and Services, 2nd ed. *Donald E. Gelfand*

Vol. 9 **Old Age on the New Scene** *Robert Kastenbaum, with 29 contributors*

Vol. 10 **Controversial Issues in Gerontology** *Harold J. Wershow, with 36 contributors*

Vol. 11 **Open Care for the Aging:** Comparative International Approaches *Virginia C. Little*

Vol. 12 **The Older Person as a Mental Health Worker** *Rosemary McCaslin, with 11 contributors*

Vol. 13 **The Elderly in Rural Society:** Every Fourth Elder *Raymond T. Coward and Gary R. Lee, with 16 contributors*

Vol. 14 **Social Support Networks and the Care of the Elderly:** Theory, Research, and Practice *William J. Sauer and Raymond T. Coward, with 17 contributors*

Vol. 15 **Managing Home Care for the Elderly:** Lessons from Community-Based Agencies *Anabel O. Pelham and William F. Clark, with 10 contributors*

Vol. 16 **A Basic Guide to Working with Elders** *Michael J. Salamon*

Vol. 17 **Communication Skills for Working with Elders** *Barbara Bender Dreher*

Vol. 18 **Ethnic Dimensions of Aging** *Donald E. Gelfand and Charles M. Barresi, with 22 contributors*

Vol. 19 **Exercise Activities for the Elderly** *Kay Flatten, Barbara Wilhite, and Eleanor Reyes-Watson*

Vol. 20 **Recreation Activities for the Elderly** *Kay Flatten, Barbara Wilhite, and Eleanor Reyes-Watson*

Vol. 21 **The Facts on Aging Quiz** *Erdman B. Palmore*

Kay Flatten was born in Kansas City and lived and studied in Topeka, Kansas, earning a B.Ed. from Washburn University of Topeka. In 1967, she entered Indiana University and began studying human movement in the field of biomechanics. She received M.S. and P.E.D. degrees, and went on to teach at the University of Wisconsin–La Crosse, the University of Indianapolis, and most recently Iowa State University. Her interest in exercise and movement patterns of older adults developed when she cared for her grandmother. Dr. Flatten now teaches courses on human movement and aging and she coordinates the undergraduate gerontology minor at Iowa State University. She and Dr. Wilhite consult on the use of the Exercise Activities and Recreation Activities for the Elderly concept and materials in various settings.

Barbara Wilhite, Ed.D., a native of Atlanta, Georgia, holds advanced degrees in Recreation and Special Education. She earned a Certificate in Gerontology from the University of Georgia. Her area of interest is therapeutic recreation and she is currently certified as a Therapeutic Recreation Specialist by the National Council for Therapeutic Recreation Certification. Her practical experiences include working with juvenile offenders, individuals with physical and mental disabilities, individuals with psychological impairments, and older adults. She has worked in both the community and institutional setting. She currently teaches within the Department of Recreation, Southern Illinois University, Carbondale. Dr. Wilhite is active in various professional organizations related to gerontology and recreation and often shares her expertise through workshops and presentations.

Eleanor Reyes-Watson was born in the Philippines and educated there and in the U.S. She received a B.Ed. from Purdue University and B.A. and M.A. degrees from the University of Wyoming. Studies in dance and an interest in the elderly led to her work with senior citizens, for several years, in a special program in St. Paul, Minnesota. In 1984, she responded to a request to develop materials for friendly visiting. While writing *Exercise Activities for the Elderly*, she studied in the Gerontology Program at Iowa State University. She is currently the volunteer coordinator for the Octagon Center for the Arts in Ames, Iowa.

Exercise Activities for the Elderly

Kay Flatten, P.E.D.
Barbara Wilhite, Ed.D.
Eleanor Reyes-Watson, M.A.

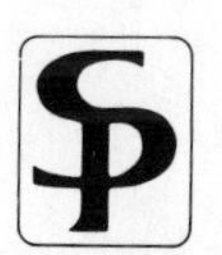

SPRINGER PUBLISHING COMPANY
NEW YORK

Springer Publishing Company, Inc.
536 Broadway
New York, NY 10012

88 89 90 91 92 / 5 4 3 2 1

Library of Congress Cataloging-in-Publication Data

Flatten, Kay.
Exercise activities for the elderly / Kay Flatten, Barbara Wilhite, Eleanor Reyes-Watson.
p. cm.
Companion v. to: Recreation activities for the elderly / Kay Flatten, Barbara Wilhite, Eleanor Reyes-Watson.
Includes bibliographies and index.
ISBN 0-8261-5910-9 (pbk.)
1. Exercise for the aged. I. Wilhite, Barbara Cathryn, 1952– . II. Flatten, Kay. III. Reyes-Watson, Eleanor. Recreation activities for the elderly. IV. Title.
[DNLM: 1. Exercise Therapy—in old age. 2. Exertion—in old age. WB 541 F586e]
GV482.6.F53 1988
613.7'0880564—dc19
DNLM/DLC
for Library of Congress 87-32139
CIP

Printed in the United States of America

Contents

APPENDICES

Preface

This book began at the request of social service agency professionals delivering programs to elderly populations. These agency professionals were involved in the delivery of nutritional and medical services to many older persons, but they felt the psychological needs of "fun and friendship" were not being adequately addressed. They were especially concerned about the lack of social contact among people who seldom leave their residences, regardless of the reason. This concern--and the ensuing request for program materials to meet this concern--were directed to Drs. Barbara Wilhite and Kay Flatten, specialists in recreation and exercises for older populations.

The intent of the program was: (1) to attract committed persons for one-on-one contact with older individuals; (2) to train these leaders in specific encounter techniques and structured activities suitable for special populations; (3) to continue to motivate these service providers to work with the frail elderly on a regular basis. Once in the leadership role, the goal was to direct the time to mutually enjoyable activities and avoid prolonged conversation on negative aspects of the older person's current situation.

The program includes training material for use by professionals in the gerontology field, directors of volunteer programs in various settings, and community or institutional exercise and recreation specialists. In addition, both volumes--Exercise Activities for the Elderly and Recreation Activities for the Elderly--give specific activity plans for use in working with frail elderly.

The program can be used by educators and social service providers alike. Colleges with gerontology curricula can use the program as a laboratory for learning about the needs and characteristics of frail elderly. Agencies offering friendly visiting can use the program to supplement their activities. Professional staff in residential care settings can add these activities to their existing recreation and exercise programming.

The authors wish to thank Ann Charles and Bev Kruempel for planting the seed of the original concept. Elizabeth Smith, Susan Scott, Faye Burke, Liz Selk, Barb Wacker, Elaine James, and Faith Balch were invaluable in trying out the original concept within their various professional capacities. Helping to put the concept on paper were Charm Price, Nancy Spiess, Janet Rickey, Darrell Simmermaker, Barb Wing, Rob Watson, and Hilary Matheson. Gratitude and respect are felt for our professional colleagues, Dr. Charles Daniel, Dr. Everett Smith, Dr. David Corbin, Dr. Helen Knierim, Dr. Janet MacLean, Dr. Rosabel Koss, Janet Pomeroy, Bernice Bateson, Dr. Helen Mills, and Dr. Helen LeBaron Hilton, who were generous with their time and critical insight in reviewing the program prior to field testing.

We have been fortunate in receiving timely support from the Department of Health and Human Services, Administration on Aging, to study further the homebound elderly and design appropriate program intervention. This support allowed the materials to be field-tested in three communities, with extensive evaluation of their impact on frail elderly, volunteer leaders, and human service agencies. In addition, the Department of Physical Education and Leisure Studies and the Research Institute for Studies in Education at Iowa State University and the Department of Recreation at Southern Illinois University provided support and encouragement to the authors. Special thanks go to Mr. William Whipple and the Hall Foundation of Cedar Rapids, Iowa, who also funded a portion of the project development costs.

Finally, we wish to thank the senior volunteers and home-centered elderly who have touched our lives, and in so doing have made this program a process of love and mutual friendship for all.

Introduction

> We must love what we are, or else we doom
> The sovereign self of slavery and hate.
> Yet, love we must the what we may become
> Lest self-indulgence substitute for fate
> And wall us up in such a tiny room
> That sun can shed no warmth, early or late.
>
> --Will C. Jumper*

WHAT IS THE EXERCISE PROGRAM?

This manual is one of a two-volume set that includes a companion book, Recreation Activities for the Elderly. Both books are designed to be used by staff or volunteers and their directors when preparing to deliver the activities to frail older persons.

Part I of each volume includes information needed to prepare the leader to use the activities. This knowledge base addresses the characteristics and needs of a frail elderly person, as well as leadership techniques and methods for working with such individuals. Basic information about exercise and physical assessment are also included in Part I. Likewise, information on recreation theory is found in Part I of Recreation Activities for the Elderly.

Part II of each book presents the activities. These are organized into interest areas (units). There are nine activity plans for each interest area, which can be used in sequence to provide continuity to the unit. Each activity plan is named and includes the purpose of the activity, the benefits of the activity, and complete directions on how to prepare for and lead the activity. References and resources

*Jumper, Will C. From time remembered. Orange, California: Foothills Press, 1977, p. 37.

are listed at the end of each unit to allow the reader to enrich his/her knowledge in the area.

A unique feature of the program is contained in the common activity plans. Each exercise unit will begin with the same "get acquainted" activity plan (Activity Plan 1) to help the leader assess the initial physical functioning level of the elder. Each unit will conclude with a community resource referral activity plan (Activity Plan 11). During this session the leader will inform the elder about services and programs in the community which may be of use in pursuing the unit topic or in maintaining self-sufficiency.

WHERE CAN THE EXERCISE PROGRAM BE USED?

There are three logical settings for the program. These range from friendly visiting in home settings to hospital, nursing home, and other institutional programs, and finally to university curricula. The program was originally designed as a resource for the Retired Senior Volunteer Program (RSVP) Friendly Visiting Programs. RSVP is a program under ACTION, established in 1969 to help older Americans take advantage of opportunities for voluntary service in their communities. The purposes of RSVP include mobilization of a large potential volunteer force, the provision of meaningful roles for retired persons, and the correction of stereotypes about older people.

Studies regarding the benefits gained by home-centered elderly through friendly visiting programs have been conducted. Tendencies for improvement in life satisfaction, perceived health status, and social isolation were found when home visits were received over an extended period. Friendly visitor programs can be a vital link between the isolated elderly and community services available for their physical, mental, and social welfare. In addition, if visitors are trained to recognize signs of stress in aged persons in their own homes, the program may prevent a crisis that would lead to relocation of the aged person--a stress which is fatal to many elderly persons.

The exercise activities in this manual can contribute to the impact of home visits. Physical exercise, even without the cardiovascular training effect, provides potential benefits to elderly participants in the areas of improved muscular strength, maintenance of bone mass, and range of joint motion. These are important factors in moving confidently within one's own environment. Exercise program materials developed for use by paraprofessionals during home visits strengthen friendly visiting programs by providing meaningful content as well as structure. These materials can direct visitation time away from conversations about losses toward positive, self-improving activities.

The exercise program can also be a part of the services provided by hospitals, nursing homes, and other residential settings. In such cases the service providers may be volunteers, as described earlier, or activities may be led by staff or family members. Since the materials are designed to be used in a one-to-one format, staff/client ratios may not allow for 1-hour sessions per client per week. In order to offer this basic contact, staff may want to train family members to deliver the program. Families have a strong desire to help, and visiting loved ones in an institutional setting can become difficult when the stay is extended. Eventually families exhaust all ideas and conversations. "How are you feeling" only goes so far, and the resident does not have a variety of experiences once the daily routine has been shared. Paid staff can offer training to family and volunteers at various times to accommodate working visitors, and can prepare a brochure to give family members upon admission of the resident.

Universities are increasing the number of courses designed to help students prepare for careers in gerontology. These recreation and exercise programs can be adapted for use in such curricula, and the manuals used as texts for such courses. Students could meet twice weekly for 1 hour to complete training in 4 weeks. Students would then be matched with elderly persons to visit once a week. The class would continue to meet once a week for the remaining 12 weeks of the semester. These class sessions would be used to discuss experiences and continue with learning activities.

The instructor can assign the units to students and establish a resource library for the students to use in conducting sessions. Students and instructor can work together to plan a party at the end of the semester.

An interesting adaptation of this course is to invite well elderly to enroll. In this way a college student can have experience working with two levels of aging, the well elderly, still in the mainstream of society, and the frail elderly.

WHO ARE THE LEADERS OF THE EXERCISE PROGRAM?

Recreation and exercise activities are a logical extension of social services as presently provided. The best service delivery model seems to involve volunteers and leaders working within already existing networks of service to the elderly.

A survey conducted by the Bureau of Census for the federal agency for volunteerism, ACTION, has revealed that about 7 million persons aged 55 and older were engaged in volunteer work. One out of every 5 persons aged 55 to 64, and 1 out of 7 aged 65 and older contributed an average of 8 hours of service weekly to volunteer activities in their communities. The value of these services is estimated to be $11.6 billion. With current government budgetary cutbacks, the volunteer segment of our society plays a crucial role in servicing frail elderly. This is especially necessary when the delivered service is free.

Using a 1985 homemaker hourly wage rate of $10.54 from a not-for-profit visiting nurse association in Ames, Iowa, it is possible to calculate the cost in salary alone to deliver one recreation and exercise unit. The time commitment for one unit would include the following:

Hours	Breakdown
8	8 hours training
12	1-hour session for 12 weeks
12	1-hour weekly meeting of leaders for 12 weeks
6	1/2-hour preparation for each of the activity sessions
38	total hours
$10.54	hourly rate
$400.52	cost for training and leading one unit

Since training is not required before every unit, the cost to deliver subsequent units would be less. The annual cost for one leader to deliver the program would be $1,349.12. The value and worth of a volunteer leader is substantiated by these cost estimates.

This program can be adapted for use by other service recipients for all ages, such as the developmentally disabled and the chronically ill. The program can also be used in different settings, such as extended-care facilities and community leisure service organizations. Volunteers may also represent various ages and backgrounds. One such recommendation is the use of these activities in an intergenerational program.

Regardless of how closely the training and activity materials and the service delivery approach are followed, the underlying goals of the program should not be compromised. These goals are:

- to provide physical and mental well-being through fun and enjoyment;
- to maintain maximum independence and integration into the community;
- to provide feelings of self-worth to the leader and elder; and
- to direct activity time away from conversations about losses toward positive, self-improving activities.

UNIT DESCRIPTIONS

Exercises for Strength - This unit consists of a series of exercises designed to work specific joints and muscles. An accompanying manual shows the leader and elder what the exercises look like when performed, and also which muscles are strengthened. The exercises begin on an easy level and move to higher levels of difficulty with each session. The number of repetitions and the difficulty of the exercises are noted on each activity plan. The elder records progress during the unit.

Exercises for Arthritis, Diabetes, and Parkinson's Disease - Lack of activity sometimes leads to complications, especially among those who have chronic conditions. The gentle exercises in this unit encourage the nonactive individual to move, stretch, and improve breathing. The goal of the unit is to improve flexibility and prevent loss of muscle strength, while learning how to manage the target conditions.

Exercises for Special Purposes - Activities in this unit are designed to help maintain the flexibility needed to carry out tasks of daily living. Mild exercises for the neck, hands, arms, shoulders, legs, and feet are included, as well as exercises to do in bed when confined. Two special sessions are devoted to strengthening the internal muscles that help in breathing and bladder control.

The following describes units which may be found in the accompanying volume Recreation Activities for the Elderly.

Crafts - The craft activities presented in this unit are mainly of the construction type, involving the use of materials. The activities are nontechnical, inexpensive, and easily completed within one or two visits. Sample craft projects include: bread dough art and sock doll projects.

Games - The games presented in this unit range from pencil and paper and table games to modified versions of shuffleboard and golf. Some emphasize mental activities, while others are more physical.

Hobbies - This unit contains discussions on a variety of ways to pursue activities providing personal satisfaction and pleasure. Various art, reading, and craft activities presented in other units are expanded upon in this unit. Sample hobbies include: puzzles, music appreciation, astronomy, gardening, and bird watching.

Literature - This unit contains a variety of passive activities involving reading and writing skills. Examples of activities include: book reviewing, poetry reading and writing, letter writing, crossword puzzles, reading aloud, word games, and the creation of a personal scrapbook.

Remembering the Past - This unit is ideal for use when participants resist structured activity. Each session has a brief reading from a senior's autobiography. The sessions focus on topics including school days, jobs, medical remedies, and travel. The unit culminates with the making of a book about the elder's discussions during the unit.

PART I

Using the Activities Effectively

CHAPTER 1

Characteristics and Needs of the Elderly

Said the little boy, "Sometimes I drop my spoon."
Said the little old man, "I do that too."
The little boy whispered, "I wet my pants."
"I do that too," laughed the little old man.
Said the little boy, "I often cry."
The old man nodded, "So do I."
"But worst of all," said the boy, "it seems
Grown-ups don't pay attention to me."
And he felt the warmth of a wrinkled old hand.
"I know what you mean," said the little old man.

--Shel Silverstein

UNDERSTANDING AGING

One of the first questions that probably occurs to a leader is "Why is this person frail?" The older person may be experiencing one or more problems associated with being confined to the home or institution. Being familiar with these characteristics will help the leader determine the needs of the elder and make the activity more helpful and enjoyable. Aging is a universal experience and the process results in changes which have a strong impact on various aspects of a person's life. How an individual adapts to change can be crucial to emotional and physical well-being. The following concerns are the result of the normal aging process or are some common reasons elderly people are frail.

1. Sensory Loss or Decline

Some problems of the frail elderly are directly related to changes in the ability to see, hear, taste, smell, touch. Because the senses are a person's link with the outside world, they are crucial to how one perceives others and the outside world and vice versa.

2. Slower Reaction Time

Reaction time increases as a person ages, but reaction time for simple tasks does not increase as much as reaction time for complicated tasks.

3. Tendency to Fatigue

The tendency to fatigue easily may be the result of several factors. Prolonged or sudden illness, emotional stress, worry, and the like all put a strain on a person's body. Inactivity is sometimes necessary for healing, but too much inactivity results in a weakened body. Activity of a proper intensity can be extremely beneficial both physically and mentally. Becoming involved in an activity that will take the focus away from a person's usual routine or problems can be a relief and a reassurance that one still has the capacity to do, think, and feel.

4. Chronic Illness

Even though a majority of older people have few restrictions on their general activity level, most do have some kind of chronic problem during old age. The problems, however, are minor or the person learns to adjust to them. Chronic conditions that most commonly affect the aged are

arthritis
heart conditions
high blood pressure (or hypertension)
visual and hearing problems
osteoporosis
loss of teeth
aphasia (speech disorder due to brain cell damage)
diabetes
asthma and emphysema
memory and attention span declines
cancer
Parkinson's disease

Chronic illness may affect people in a variety of ways. Problems with hearing and vision, lack of strength, coordination and flexibility all limit the ability to move. Lack of mobility has an impact on the ability to take care of daily needs. Contact with other people may become more limited. Sometimes the overall effect of multiple long-term chronic illnesses is emotional problems which make it difficult to function normally.

5. Acute Illness

Examples of acute illnesses are: the flu, a cold, a cut, or a broken bone, etc. When an older person has an acute illness, the impact can often be severe. For example, when an older person receives a cut, there is greater chance of infection because of reduced circulation. A disorder such as flu can be serious for somone who does not have the reserve capacity to fight it off. Acute illness may have the effect of causing a person to be temporarily bedridden, disrupting daily routines and requiring assistance with daily tasks.

6. Lack of Transportation

Mobility outside the home is very important to a person's sense of independence. Lack of transportation makes it difficult to provide for one's needs and forces one to depend on others to satisfy those needs. This may result in feelings of frustration, resentment, and isolation.

Some of the reasons for lack of transportation include limited finances, living in an area that is not serviced by a public transportation system, or having a disability that makes it difficult to travel without the aid of specially equipped vehicles.

7. Emotional Sensitivity

Emotionally related problems include the loss of roles such as that of a spouse, mother, sibling, friend, or professional, and the loss of loved ones. For many older people, fear limits involvement. Feeling safe in one's environment adds incentive to become involved in the community.

8. Financial Problems

Many older people live on limited or fixed incomes. Today money buys many things--even good health. Limited income can affect a person's mental and emotional well-being. Participation in some social events or educational activities, such as travel, special classes, lectures, and concerts, is sometimes limited by finances.

NEEDS OF THE ELDERLY

Understanding the characteristics common to frail elderly individuals will be helpful in identifying their needs. In general, these needs can be grouped as physical, social, intellectual, emotional, or spiritual. Needs that can be specifically addressed by the exercise program are:

- (a) the need to continue using body muscles and joints to prevent loss of strength and flexibility;
- (b) the need to feel safe and secure while carrying out physical activities;
- (c) the need to maintain contact with a variety of people;
- (d) the need to maintain and acquire friends;
- (e) the need for opportunities to learn new skills and develop new interests;

(f) the need to maintain self-esteem; and
(g) the need to feel useful.

To test your knowledge of the characteristics of the elderly and to point out potential prejudices in your perceptions of older persons, complete the following quiz. Answers for the quiz can be found on page 10.

QUIZ ON ATTITUDES ABOUT AGING*

VISION

T F Cataracts are common among older people.

T F The older people become, the poorer their eyesight.

T F Glasses can always help older people see better.

T F Accidents can be related to vision problems in older people.

T F Older people prefer duller colors than do younger people.

T F Many experts feel that the lens of the eye yellows with age.

HEARING

T F If an older person is hard of hearing, you should speak louder to be heard.

T F If people have hearing aids, they can usually hear what you are saying.

T F Having people read your lips as you are talking helps them to understand what you are saying.

T F If people who are hard of hearing do not see you, you should find some way to let them know you are in the room.

T F Older people usually know if they have a hearing problem.

T F Hearing loss frequently occurs in both ears.

*Adapted from Ernst, M., & Shore, H. Sensitizing people to the process of aging: The in-service educator's guide. Denton, TX: Dallas Geriatric Research Institute, 1977.

TACTILE

T F Touching people helps them to understand what you are saying.

T F Most older people do not like to be touched.

T F Older people sometimes develop blisters on their feet without noticing them.

T F Many times burns are caused because people do not notice the heat until it is too late.

T F Strokes, arthritis, and Parkinson's disease can all affect a person's ability to hold or to feel objects.

T F If people have lost their touch perception, there is little that anyone can do to help them.

DEXTERITY

T F Older people may spill their coffee because they cannot grip the cup.

T F Counting change is very easy for older people.

T F Threading a needle takes a lot of coordination.

T F Few older people suffer from decreased ability to hold objects.

T F If people have difficulty dressing or feeding themselves, it is better for someone to do it for them in order to save time.

T F People with dexterity problems find small objects easier to handle than large objects.

TASTE

T F People's appetites change throughout life.

T F Older people often use more seasonings on their food than they did when they were younger.

T F Salty food can be harmful to the elderly.

T F Older people often complain about the way food tastes.

T F Older people can taste sweets better than other foods.

T F If people must be fed by other persons, it does not really matter to them what they are eating.

SMELL

T F Body odor is a common problem among older people.

T F The ability to smell odors does not change with age.

T F Older people can smell smoke as well as anyone.

T F Smell is important to the taste of food.

T F Older people do not notice bad odors as quickly as other people.

T F When working around older people, staff should wear strong perfume or shaving lotion so that the older person can smell it.

MOBILITY AND BALANCE

T F Most older people will end up in wheelchairs.

T F Falling down is a big problem for older people.

T F Joints which are not used tend to get stiff.

T F Younger people have dizzy spells more often than older people do.

T F The major reasons that older people walk slowly is that they cannot think very well.

T F Some medications can affect a person's mobility and balance.

GENERAL

T F An older person can still contribute to society.

T F A person is old when he reaches age 65.

T F All people 60 years old are in the same physical condition.

T F As people get older, they become less intelligent.

T F Most older people live in hospitals, nursing homes, homes for the aged, or other institutions.

T F Most older people are interested in learning new things when they are given the chance.

REFERENCES AND RESOURCES

ACTION. The value of volunteer services in the United States. Pamphlet #3530.4, Stock #0456-000-00015-1, 1976. Washington, DC: U.S. Government Printing Office.

Birren, J. E., & Schaie, K. W. (Eds.). Handbook of the psychology of aging. New York: Van Nostrand Reinhold, 1977.

Bogart, A. G., & Larson, L. An evaluation of two visiting programs for elderly community residents. International Journal of Aging and Human Development, 1983; 17(4), 267-279.

Carroll, K. (Ed.). Compensating for sensory loss. Minneapolis, MN: Ebenezer Center for Aging and Human Development, 1978.

Crandall, R. C. Gerontology: A behavioral science approach. Reading, MA: Addison-Wesley, 1980.

Cummings, E., & Henry, W. In L. Troll (Ed.), Continuations: Adult development and aging. Monterey, CA: Brooks/Cole, 1982.

Ernst, M., & Shore, H. Sensitizing people to the processes of aging: The in-service educator's guide. Denton, TX: Dallas Geriatric Research Institute, 1977.

Jarvick, L. F. (Ed.). Aging into the 21st century. New York: Gardner Press, 1978.

Jumper, W. C. From time remembered. Orange, CA: Foothills Press, 1977.

Morris, W. W., & Hades, I. M. (Eds.). Hoffman's daily needs and interests of older people. Springfield, IL: Charles C. Thomas, 1983.

Mulligan, M. A., & Bennett, R. Development and evaluation of a friendly visitor program for the community aged. International Journal of Aging and Human Development, 1977; 8(1), 43-66.

National Council on the Aging. Fact book on aging: A profile of America's older population. Washington, DC: NCDA Research and Evaluation Department, 1978.

_____. Working with the at-risk older person: A resource manual. Washington, DC: NCDA, 1981.

Retired Senior Volunteer Program: Operation handbook. No. 4405.92, August, 1983. Washington, DC: U.S. Government Printing Office.

Silverstein, S. A light in the attic. New York: Harper & Row, 1981. Copyright ©1981 by Evil Eye Music, Inc. Reprinted by permission of Harper & Row, Publishers, Inc.

Smith, E. L. The aging process and benefits of physical activities. In <u>Research and practical activity programs for the aging</u>. Pre-convention Symposium and Workshop Papers, American Alliance of Health, Physical Education, Recreation, and Dance, 1982.

Troll, L. E. <u>Continuations: Adult development and aging</u>. Monterey, CA: Brooks/Cole, 1982.

U.S. Department of Health, Education and Welfare. <u>Working with older people: A guide to practice</u>, vol. 1. Rockville, MD: U.S. Government Printing Office, 1978.

U.S. Public Health Service, Health Resource Administration. <u>Limitations of activity and mobility due to chronic conditions</u>. Vital and Health Statistics, Data from the National Health Series 10, No. 96. DHEW (HRA)75-1523. Rockville, MD: National Center for Health Statistics, 1974.

Key to the Quiz on Page 6.

VISION	HEARING
T, T, F, T, F, T	F, F, T, T, F, F
TACTILE	**DEXTERITY**
T, F, T, T, T, F	T, F, T, F, F, F
TASTE	**SMELL**
T, T, T, T, F, F	T, F, F, T, T, F
MOBILITY AND BALANCE	**GENERAL**
F, T, T, F, F, T	T, F, F, F, F, T

CHAPTER 2
Learning About Exercises

> If exercise could be packed into a pill, it would be the single most widely prescribed, and beneficial medicine in the nation.
>
> --Norman Butler

This chapter includes information needed in order to lead exercise activities. The importance of different kinds of exercises and various body positions during exercise is noted. Chronic conditions which limit exercise are explained, and those conditions benefiting from exercise are presented. The reader will learn how the medical profession views exercise for seniors and how an exercise leader works with physicians. Information about conducting exercise sessions using the activities is also included.

THE ROLE OF THE PHYSICIAN

The physician is important in screening exercises for older adults. Before beginning an exercise activity, take the specific exercise unit to the elder's doctor and leave it for evaluation. When a doctor can see the pictures and read the description of a specific exercise, an appropriate decision can be made for the patient. Remember to ask if there is a charge for such a screening. If so, it is best cleared with the elder first. One may choose to mail the exercise unit to the physician and return later to pick it up.

If the physician does not want his/her patient to exercise, then a unit from the companion book Recreation Activities for the Elderly (Flatten, Wilhite, & Reyes-Watson; also available from Springer Publishing Co.) can be selected. To exercise without physician approval is to act irresponsibly and could endanger the well-being of the elder as well as lead to liability problems.

While the exercise activities are being reviewed, the leader and elder can spend their activity time on the tests of physical functioning. Two flexibility tests and one strength test are presented on pages 35 to 39, and an activity plan for their use is included in Chapter 5 (pages 45 through 47).

When interacting with the physician, realize that until recently, the medical prescription for heart attack rehabilitation was complete bed rest. Medical schools are just beginning to emphasize geriatric medicine and exercise physiology. The result of this transition is that some physicians prescribe exercise and encourage activity in their recovering or chronically ill patients, while others get upset at the word "exercise" and tell their patients to take it easy until they feel like doing activity. This latter approach usually results in no attempt to exercise.

A third group of physicians is knowledgeable about exercise and supportive of it for their patients but skeptical about exercise programs in the community. When they are asked to sign permission slips for patients to join an exercise class, they may not sign because they have no idea what form the exercise will take. Understanding the various kinds of exercise and communicating the nature of those used in the program to the physician and elder is an important starting point.

KINDS OF EXERCISE

How the body is positioned has a direct effect on which muscles are used in exercise. Here are some rules of thumb concerning the relationship of body position and gravity.

Sitting is more stable than standing, as gravity is less likely to cause one to topple in a chair. Seated positions usually work upper body muscles.

Standing positions are the most strenuous because the heart must work harder and because the individual is supporting and moving the entire body weight. These positions usually work lower body muscles and back muscles.

Lying positions are the easiest because the heart need not work to pump the blood upward and because the majority of the body weight is supported. These positions can use the greatest number of muscles; however, a person must do exercises while on the stomach, back, right side, and left side.

The three body positions, lying, sitting, and standing, use different muscles. A good exercise program should use all three positions if possible.

Regardless of body position, the exercises most commonly performed by seniors are slow, easy movements using full joint range of motion. Such exercises are used frequently in this book. Typically, a person sits in a chair and moves fingers, forearms, arms, feet, or calves in a flexing, then straightening manner. Many such exercises include slow circling actions at a particular joint, such as circling each finger or circling arms in a slow swimming action resembling the back-crawl or the front-crawl. People often do such exercises to music in 3/4 or 4/4 time and move on the first beat of each measure. An example would be "Reach for the ceiling -2-3-4, reach for the floor -2-3-4," or "Look to the right -2-3-4, look to the left -2-3-4."

Such exercises are designed to increase range of joint motion in the joint moved. Moving a joint through its entire range several times is good for the joint, especially if the joint is arthritic. Range can be restored in a joint after surgery by such exercises.

There is a saying, "use it or lose it," and this is very true of joint range of motion. Age has been found to decrease flexibility, and older people say they feel better when they are "stretched out." These slow, weightless exercises do very little to develop muscular strength, as the muscles must work only against the weight of the limb. Since most of these exercises are done while sitting in a chair, the weight of the upper body limbs is not enough to develop strength.

Muscle strength can, however, be developed in the lower body by such exercises. The weight of the entire leg is enough to strengthen muscular tissue; also, lifting the body weight by rising from a chair or doing knee bends will develop leg strength.

Because the weight of the body, or the legs, is significant, many extremely frail persons cannot do some of the exercises in this book. Even if people can do these exercises, care must be taken not to place a strain on the heart.

Exercises with slow, easy movements represent the simplest form of exercise when done from a seated position. They contribute to range of motion in the joint; however, they do not add much to muscular strength and add nothing to cardiovascular functioning. Standing exercises moving the leg or whole body, or seated exercises moving one or both legs, do develop strength in the lower body. Most exercise programs begin with this type of exercise because it places the least stress on the body. The leader can watch the frail person's response to such easy movements before adding other forms of exercise.

A more advanced form of exercise found in this book is very similar to what has been described above; however, there is something added to the exercise. That something has either weight or elasticity. It can be a plastic bottle (with a handle) partially filled with water, or a can of food, or a rubber tube. The object has the ability to increase the muscle strength required to move it.

These exercises give all the benefits of the previous exercises as well as the benefit of muscle strength development in the upper body. Because there is an increased demand on the muscles, a greater need exists to watch for cardiovascular stress. If a person has difficulty doing slow, easy movements using a full range of motion without extra resistance, extra resistance should not be added. The exception to this would be if the difficulty stems from joint stiffness and not muscle strength or heart weakness. A stiff joint needs progressive resistance to rebuild range of motion.

It is important to understand the following three principles when doing these exercises:

1. When holding a weight in the hands or on the feet, THE FARTHER THE WEIGHT IS FROM THE JOINT, THE MORE EFFORT IS REQUIRED TO MOVE THE LIMB AND WEIGHT. To make the exercise easier, move the weight closer to the joint.

2. When stretching a tube, the thicker the diameter and the shorter the tube, the more resistance it has. Bicycle inner tubes which are 27 inches by 1¼ inches or 1½ inches are very good for mild resistance. HOLDING A TUBE SO AS TO SHORTEN IT WILL MAKE THE EXERCISE MORE DIFFICULT.

3. Never produce so much resistance that a person has muscle soreness the next day. It is best to BUILD STRENGTH WITHOUT SORENESS.

Another kind of exercise is done with rapid movements. Such exercise is dangerous for frail older persons and consequently is not included in this program. Adding to the problem is the fact that this form of exercise is what people usually think of when the word "exercise" is mentioned. These exercises can be as already described but with the rate of repetition increased. If done to music, as in aerobic dance, a movement is made on every beat instead of every fourth beat. The rhythm would be "reach (1), reach (2), reach (3), reach (4)" or "kick (1), kick (2), kick (3), kick (4)."

Exercises of any kind done rapidly cause the heart to work harder to supply oxygen to the working muscles at a faster rate. Even though this is a good way to strengthen the heart and improve cardiovascular function, the exercises in this book are not likely to be supervised by exercise leaders trained to work on cardiovascular fitness. Therefore, EXERCISES IN THIS PROGRAM SHOULD NEVER BE DONE RAPIDLY OR CONTINUED IF SIGNS OF INCREASED BREATHING, FLUSHING, OR SWEATING OCCUR.

Exercises done at a rapid rate have two disadvantages: first, they cause a response of the cardiovascular system, which the activities in this book avoid; and second, they result in "throwing" the limb. The limb keeps going on its own (using momentum) without requiring muscles.

The specific cardiovascular responses that will occur within the second minute of a workout using rapid movements are:

increased heart rate

increased blood pressure

increased cardiac output (amount of blood leaving the heart per beat)

increased breathing rate

And within 5 minutes the following will occur:

flushing of the skin

sweating

increased depth in each breath

Other exercises that cause such cardiovascular responses include jogging, bicycling, swimming, rope jumping, stair climbing, even walking if done briskly. IT IS VERY IMPORTANT FOR OLDER PEOPLE DOING SUCH EXERCISES TO HAVE AN EXAMINATION BY A CARDIOLOGIST BEFORE BEGINNING SUCH A PROGRAM. If any participant in the program, leader or elder, notices one or more of the seven physical responses listed above while performing a workout, he/she should stop the exercise immediately.

BENEFITS REALIZED AFTER AN EXERCISE PROGRAM

The benefits gained by an exercise program depend on three factors: the intensity of the workout, the duration of the workout, and the number of workouts per week. Workouts lasting at least 20 minutes and occurring at least three times per week are the minimum for gaining benefits from exercise. The intensity depends on the individual. To some, lifting one leg will be enough of an overload to bring about strength gains; others may require extra weight at the ankle to get strength gains. It is always better with a frail person to underestimate the person's proper intensity level. This is less effective for achieving benefits, but it is safer. Remember, a person can start at a low intensity and increase as the program progresses. This provides both safety and psychological advantages. Adding a little resistance shows growth and improvement.

Exercises in this program have been specifically written to eliminate any cardiovascular stress. This means that changes in the heart and blood vessels will not take place. However, joint range of motion should improve, and muscular strength may improve. Both of these play a major role in performing activities of daily living. Being able to move one's own body from the bed to a chair, in and out of the bathtub, and up stairs is basic to living alone safely.

The nature of the exercise program limits the physical benefits that can be expected: (1) the materials provide no cardiovascular activities; (2) the leader works with the elder once a week (two short of the number of desired workouts); and (3) the intensity is expected to be low because of the nature of the frail elderly. Even so, gains in flexibility and self-image are possible through correct use of these materials.

CHRONIC CONDITIONS AND EXERCISE

After learning about chronic conditions, one may wonder, "Why consider exercise?" The best answer to that question is "Why not?" Movement is as necessary for a person as food and sleep. Chronic conditions do not preclude exercise. The key to the issue of illness and exercise is WHAT KIND AND HOW MUCH. Decisions on these two points depend on the chronic condition and the individual.

There is a wealth of literature in the form of free booklets about exercises for specific conditions. Also, physical therapists have exercises for musculoskeletal conditions. Some general ideas about specific conditions are presented below to show how exercise is considered important for each condition.

Arthritis--Arthritis responds well to water exercises which help relieve the effect of gravity compressing the joints. The buoyant effect of water helps relieve pressure on a joint. The resistance for strengthening muscles comes from water resistance, not gravity. In the absence of a pool, exercises should be done from a seated position.

High blood pressure and heart problems--This condition responds well to walking if the problem stems from other than genetic sources (inherited). The program exercises will not help this condition because they are not intense enough to cause a cardiovascular change.

Diabetes--Diabetes responds well to mild exercise, which helps control caloric intake and expenditure.

Reconstructed joint--Physical exercise is always prescribed after joint surgery. It is usually led by a physical therapist.

Continued exercising, as in this program, is excellent for maintaining muscle strength around the joint.

Visual impairment--Some eye problems can be helped by strengthening the small muscles of the eye. The physician knows if this is possible and has corrective exercises.

Obesity--Obesity responds well to moderate-intensity, long-duration activities done frequently. This will increase caloric expenditure and contribute to weight loss.

Incontinence--This condition responds well to Kegel exercises which are designed to strengthen the muscles around the urethra and anus.

Parkinson's disease--This condition requires exercise to maintain muscle length. Exercises that gently stretch and strengthen are best.

Lower back pain--Certain exercises such as Williams's back exercises and abdominal strengtheners help prevent lower back pain.

Mastectomy--Exercise is required after surgery and is usually given by the physician and/or physical therapist. This helps maintain range of motion of the shoulder joint.

LEADERSHIP CONCERNS

The exercise units and the training information have been written to minimize potential problems. Following the guidelines and using common sense are the two most important factors in preventing dangerous situations. Even so, the motto "expect the unexpected" is a good approach to safe leadership.

Cardiac problems are the most serious dangers to exercise leaders. That is why there is emphasis on the relationship between speed of movement and heart stress. Keep the exercises slow and pause between exercises. If any of the normal signs of increased cardiovascular activity occur--sweating, flushing, deep or rapid breathing--stop the exercise session and contact the program coordinator during the week. The coordinator will then follow up with the physician. If angina begins, stop the session and follow the above procedure. Angina is a pain in the chest caused when the heart is not getting enough oxygen to meet its work requirements.

If the participant feels lightheaded, dizzy, or nauseous, has a pain in the left arm, or has the feeling of digestive "heartburn," then immediately stop the exercise session and have the person lie down on a couch or bed. Call the doctor first, and then the program coordinator immediately. Do not try to give water or medicine unless nitroglycerin is prescribed and available. The best thing to do is to sit with the elder until medical advice or help arrives. The leader may want to make some notes during this time; for example, when problem began, symptoms, and changes.

Another consideration is the chance of falling. To prevent this, the exercises have been written to be done either from a chair or standing holding a chair. The leader must always help the elder get into a safe position before beginning an exercise. Even so, it is possible for a person to fall over in a chair or have their knees give out while standing and holding a chair. Should this happen, it is doubtful that the leader can break the fall because everything happens too quickly. The fall will be less dangerous if the person is on carpet and far from furniture with sharp corners. A safe situation should exist before each exercise session begins. If a person should fall, DO NOT TRY TO HELP HIM/HER UP. Reassure the person and encourage lying still for a while. After the elder is calm, ask if there is any pain anywhere. If there is no pain, move one limb at a time, gently. If no pain is felt, it is safe to get up. If pain exists in any joint or bone, cover the person with a blanket, call the doctor first, and then the program coordinator for advice.

The figure below illustrates the stages to follow when rising from the floor: (1) have the person crawl to a couch or chair, continue until the top half of the body is on the chair seat with the front edge of the seat in the belly button; (2) now bring one foot up under the hip, for support; (3) on the count of three, the elder pushes down on the chair seat with the arms and the floor with the tucked leg, while the leader helps lift the hips; (4) once the person has pulled the second leg up to stand on, and is leaning over the chair seat, he/she should pause for a moment to let the heart adjust to the change in body position; (5) finally, he/she turns and sits in the chair.

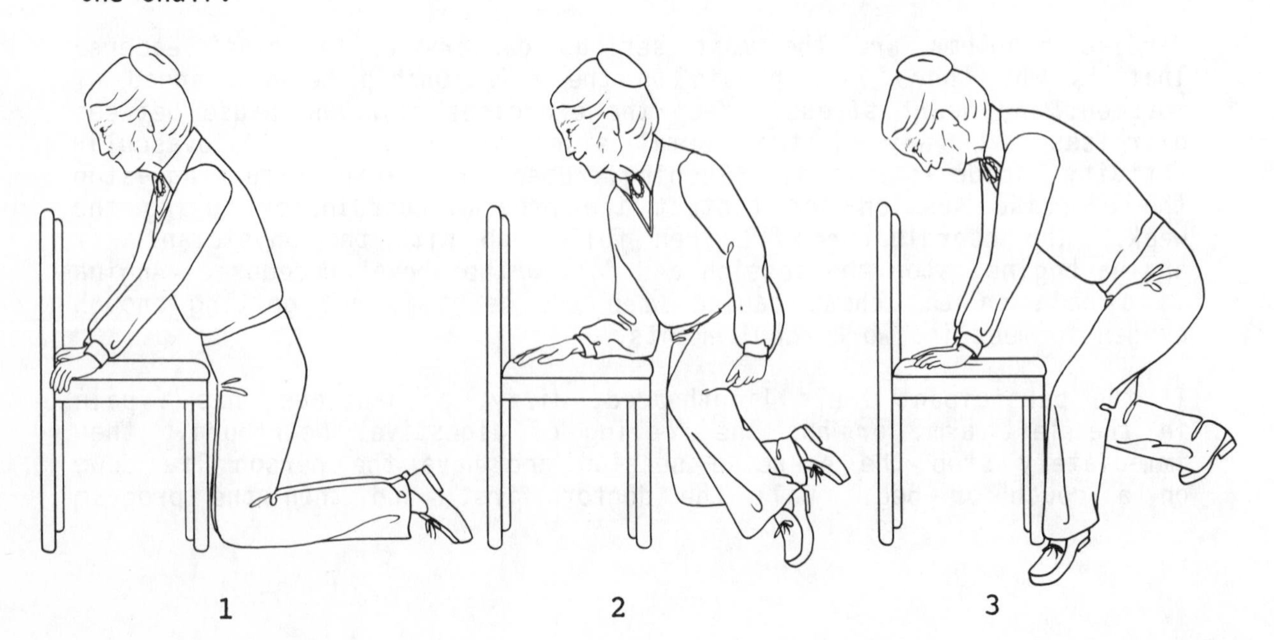

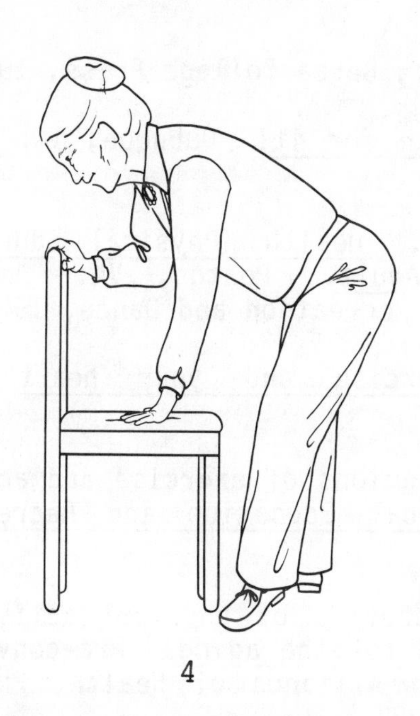

4

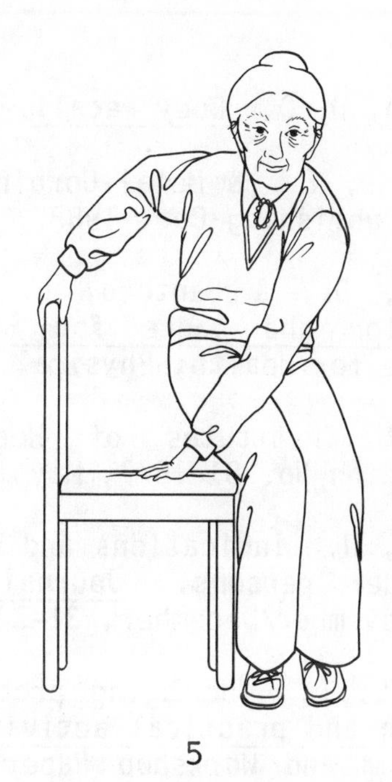

5

The safety of the exercise sessions has been maximized by design. The chances for accident and injury are small; however, the leader should be ready to respond to the following:

HEART STRESS	Stop exercise, call the physician and program coordinator if heart attack is suspected.
FALLS	Keep the person calm and still; move his/her limbs gently; call physician if pain exists; if no pain, have the person crawl to chair; help up.
MUSCULOSKELETAL PAIN	Avoid exercise and call program coordinator during the week.

Be prepared, conservative, and observant as a leader, but do not be frightened.

REFERENCES AND RESOURCES

American Alliance for Health, Physical Education, Recreation and Dance. Research and practical physical activity programs for the aged. Pre-convention Symposium and Workshop Papers, National Convention, 1982.

Butler, R. N. Public interest report No. 23: Exercise, the neglected therapy. Journal of Aging and Human Development, 1977-78; 8(2), 193-195.

Cantu, R. C. Diabetes and exercise. New York: E. P. Dutton, 1982.

Chrisman, D. C. Body recall. Berea, KY: Berea College Press, 1980.

Corbin, D. E., & Metal-Corbin, J. Reach for it! Dubuque, IA: Eddie Bowers Publishing Co., 1983.

Leviton, D., & Santoro, L. C. (Eds.). Health, Physical Education, Recreation and Dance for the Older Adult. Reston, VA: American Alliance for Health, Physical Education, Recreation and Dance, 1980.

National Institutes of Health. Exercise and your heart. NIH Publication No. 81-1677, May 1981.

Piscopo, J. Indications and contraindications of exercise and activity for older persons. Journal of Physical Education and Recreation, 1979; November/December, 31-34.

Smith, E. L. The aging process and benefits of physical activities. Research and practical activity programs for the aging. Pre-convention Symposium and Workshop Papers, American Alliance of Health, Physical Education, Recreation and Dance, 1982, 1-28.

U.S. National Center for Health Statistics. Vital and health statistics, Series 10, October-June, 1967-69, No. 40-53.

CHAPTER 3

Conducting the Activities

....the key to the success of any recreation and exercise experience is in large measure the quality of leadership. There is no substitute for good leadership.

BASIC CONCEPTS OF TEACHING AND LEARNING

To gain full enjoyment and satisfaction from the program, the participant must have at least a minimal amount of skill and knowledge of the activities. Thus, the leader's responsibilities often involve teaching. As exercises are introduced, the leader must teach the needed skills. Five basic concepts of teaching and learning are highlighted below.

1. Awareness of individual differences: Each elder is an individual and must learn in a unique way. As leaders become aware of the differences among seniors, they will avoid a standardized approach to teaching and will not expect all to learn the same things or at the same rate.

2. Learning by doing: In general, the elder will learn best by doing. This does not mean that the individual must be physically active. The nature of the doing depends on the activity. For example, learning about arthritis may involve looking at newspaper articles, a physically passive act; the individual, however, is involved in "doing."

3. Reinforcement and feedback: This important concept maintains that when the elder performs as desired, these actions should be encouraged so that they will be repeated. Once behaviors are well established, praise may be needed less often. This concept also emphasizes the importance of providing feedback to give some idea of progress. This feedback may include informing of needed corrections. The essential point is that

positive reinforcement, with appropriate feedback, results in faster and more efficient learning.

4. Importance of personal meaning: People learn best that which has, or comes to have, personal meaning. The leader should thus help the elder realize how the activity skill or knowledge being taught is personally related and what benefits will be gained by learning the activity.

5. Existing knowledge: New information will be more easily learned if it is related to what is already known. This concept requires that the leader know what the senior has already learned about an activity.

GENERAL SUGGESTIONS FOR LEADING AN ACTIVITY

The key to the success of the program will be the ability of the leader to direct a variety of activities. The following are hints to consider.

Always try to be at ease, optimistic, and positive in manner; emphasize the positive, not the negative.

Break up the activity into small parts so that it will be easier to teach. Establish smaller goals that combine into larger ones.

Identify the basic purpose/intent of the activity and give reasons (or benefits) for doing the activity.

Never promise anything on which it is not possible to follow through.

Let interest and enthusiasm be contagious. Also have fun as a leader!

Participate in the activity to the extent possible. Encourage as much involvement as possible, allowing the elder the opportunity to lead, when appropriate.

Try to foresee and eliminate unexpected barriers or conditions that may result in problems.

Treat the elder as an individual, recognizing individual values, interests, and abilities; show respect and help maintain dignity.

Do not be disappointed if there is initial suspiciousness or nonacceptance. With familiarity and trust sincerity will be accepted.

Be a good listener!

STAGES OF AN ACTIVITY SESSION

Preparing for the activity: The leader should know the activity thoroughly. Sometimes, this means practicing the activity in advance with another person or persons. Any needed equipment should be gathered and other required pre-planning as indicated on the activity plan should be performed. Also, consider the space that will be needed to accommodate the activity. It is helpful to read one activity plan beyond. This will allow the leader to check out the resources and restrictions of the environment in advance. For example, exercises done during the "In-Bed Flexibility Exercises" session require a couch or bed that is accessible to the leader and senior.

Try to prepare the elder by developing feelings of confidence about the activity. As the activity is described, try to find out what is already known; begin instruction at that point.

Explanation and demonstration: The leader should be in a position to be seen and heard. Instructions should be clear and brief but presented without rushing. The activity should be presented one step at a time. Demonstration of the activity is essential in most cases. Give the elder a chance to ask questions regarding the directions; however, try to avoid lengthy explanations. Remember, the best learning occurs during involvement; get the senior involved as soon as possible.

Encourage and support participation during every stage of the session. Think of learning as sharing and interacting rather than directing and controlling. The explanation and demonstration stage will be most meaningful when the senior has some input.

Practice: Let the elder do the activity, guiding efforts and correcting when necessary. As the activity is performed, make sure the steps and procedures are understood. Remember to provide encouragement and feedback.

Evaluation: No activity will proceed perfectly without potential for further improvement. Evaluation consists of thinking about strengths and weaknesses of the activity. The leader relies primarily on observing and writing down significant aspects of the session. The leader is thus helping to determine if the session went well and if the elder is achieving the desired benefits from the activity. Revisions can be made based on the results of evaluation.

As the activity is completed, the leader should consider the following types of questions: (1) Was the activity enjoyable? (2) Was the activity too difficult or too easy? (3) Was the activity too long for the allotted time? (4) Does the elder wish to repeat the activity? (5) Were the materials and supplies required for the activity adequate? (6) What related activities may be attempted? (7) What significant progress or behavior occurred during the activity?

Occasionally, the leader may be asked to summarize evaluation comments and report to the program coordinator. This might occur, for example, if problems were frequently encountered during activity time. The primary purpose of evaluation, however, is to help the leader learn how to make activity time as enjoyable and beneficial as possible.

UTILIZING THE ACTIVITY PLAN FORMAT

The activity session should follow the structure outlined in the activity plan format below:

ACTIVITY PLAN:

PURPOSE OF ACTIVITY:

DESCRIPTION OF ACTIVITY:

BENEFITS OF ACTIVITY:

BEFORE THE SESSION:

Things to make or do

Things to take

WHAT TO DO DURING THE SESSION:

Greeting and opening chat; pay attention to any immediate needs.

Complete any unfinished business from previous session.

Explain the session's activities.

Do activities.

Session wrap-up; enjoy a snack if desired.

ENDING THE SESSION:

Sharing the basket.

Talk about and confirm next session.

AFTER THE SESSION:

Write up comments.

IDEAS FOR MODIFYING THE ACTIVITY:

TIPS FOR SAFETY:

The activity plan begins with basic information to the leader such as a description, benefits, goals and objectives of the activity. It is important to be familiar with this basic information. The section "Before the Session" provides information regarding what the leader will need to do in preparation for the session. This section includes a listing of specific supplies and materials needed for the activity. In the third section, step-by-step instructions for conducting the activity are provided. Lastly, the activity plan includes ideas for modifying the session to meet certain needs of the elder and tips for safety.

Each session begins with a review of the activity conducted in the previous period and concludes with a preview of what will occur during the next session. This structure will assist in maintaining continuity, and is particularly helpful if problems with short-term memory are present.

It is important for the leader to take time during the beginning of each session to note the present condition of the elder. Some days will not be good days. When this occurs, do not attempt to force the planned activity, as this will prove counterproductive. It is best to reschedule the activity or conduct it during the next regularly scheduled time. Noting the present condition of the elder also provides an opportunity to detect special problems and concerns which may be referred by the sponsoring agency to other service providers such as visiting nurses, homemaker-health aids, and the like.

Providing a time to share a snack is a special feature of the activity plan. This provides a good opportunity for social interaction. It also provides an opportunity for the elder to experience a feeling of responsibility and self-worth by preparing something for the session. Snacks should be simple and healthful. The leader should be familiar with any dietary restrictions indicated for the senior. The option to delete snack time can be chosen if desired. Having a banana or apple in a tote basket when going to a session ensures the opportunity for a snack, should the elder be unprepared.

Another optional feature of the activity plan is "sharing the basket." To "share the basket," the leader must work with two frail elderly persons or work in partnership with another leader. When working with each elder, the leaders ask if there is something of interest the elder would like the leaders to take and share with another person. The leaders then place the items in their tote baskets and listen to stories or information about the items. During the week, the leaders meet and exchange items and stories. In their next session with their elders, the leaders show the items and repeat the stories. On subsequent sessions, each leader will return a shared item, explain an item from the other elder, and collect a new item of significance to share in return. In this way, the leaders serve as a means of communication between two people, which may develop further through telephoning, letter writing, and possibly, visiting. The types of items to be shared will vary. They might include pictures, postcards, souvenirs, edible items, craft items, stories, favorite sayings, jokes, trivia questions, and so on. Do not take items of great worth. The possibility of misplacing an item is always a factor to consider.

At the end of each session, preferably after the session, the leader should record any significant progress or behavior that occurred during the activity. The leader should also note particular concerns or impressions. These written comments will be helpful in preparing to work with the elder each week and may also be shared with the program coordinator, if appropriate.

LEADERSHIP METHODS IN MOTIVATION

Motivation is something that comes from within. Accordingly, the frequently used phrase "motivating an individual to participate" really means stimulating a person's own motivation to seek involvement and self-direction.

Many elders will be self-motivated to participate in activities. Others, however, will only go through the motions or will not participate at all. While the senior's desire should be respected as much as possible, an attempt should be made to stimulate interest when nonacceptance threatens overall well-being.

There are two basic ways to stimulate an individual's own motivation. One is by the nature of the activity itself. Certain activities are by nature attractive and make the individual want to participate. In cases of reluctance to participate, time should be taken to determine which activities are attractive to the elder. The second method centers on coaxing participation. In some cases, it is necessary to get the senior involved at least to the extent that certain aspects of the activity stimulate interests, resulting in motivation. Three approaches to coaxing are discussed below.

Involve the elder in many types of activities in the hopes that one of them--or an aspect of one of them--will result in motivation. This approach may be likened to "sampling," whereby a person is exposed to a variety of activities and individual preferences are noted.

Present activities that are a direct reflection of the elder's interests and/or needs. For example, Mr. Doe has a need for social interaction and has expressed an interest in reading. Thus, the leader might suggest that Mr. Doe join in a discussion concerning a book about exercise.

Other suggestions that may help to ensure successful participation are:

Try to put the elder at ease; create an accepting and supportive environment.

Take extra time to talk about needs, interests, and abilities.

Explain the program and encourage questions.

In the beginning, select activities that are most likely to succeed.

Make the elder feel as if participation is appreciated by the leader.

Give credit when it is due, but avoid flattery. A compliment on something that obviously did not turn out well can be belittling; but recognition of progress, however slight, is rewarding.

It may be necessary to allow the elder to be a spectator in the beginning; this approach may stimulate the interest and encourage future participation.

Recognize the importance of timing. Everyone travels at an individual pace and readiness for involvement will differ. Someone who has been inactive for a number of years will require much nurturing. Move slowly in directing interests and realize that participation may occur during one session and not during the next.

Plan to spend more time during the "Greeting and opening chat" section of the activities plan.

Additional time spent listening and recognizing feelings may be needed before attempting the activity. In these cases, going immediately into an activity may hinder more than help the situation.

Recognize that some days just will not be good days, and efforts to conduct the activity will not be successful. In this situation, it is probably best to "just visit," perhaps ending the session early, to reschedule for another time during the week or to conduct the activity plan during the next regularly scheduled time.

BARRIERS TO EFFECTIVE COMMUNICATION

Individuals are dependent on the ability to make their thoughts, feelings, and needs known to others. Effective communication is the result of those efforts. Communication is the sending and receiving of messages. The fact that a message was sent does not guarantee that it was received or understood.

For effective communication to be possible between any two persons, one must be aware of the conditions that may cause barriers to effective communication.

Conversation may be difficult if you are guilty of:	How to avoid these communication barriers
No eye contact	Look at the elder.
Cutting off elder	Allow the elder to finish.
Stereotyping	Do not allow appearances, body language, or what is said turn you off.
Bypassing	Respond to what the elder has said before interjecting your thoughts.
Knowing it all	Allow yourself to learn from the elder. You may not have all the answers.
Inferring	Don't assume you know what the elder has to say. Don't finish his/her sentence.
Mind wandering	Give your attention.
Defensiveness	Check out the other's intention before forming your opinion.
Hidden agenda	Help to clarify what the elder wishes to discuss so that you are both talking about the same issue.
Disinterest in needs	Listen for needs even though you also have needs to be met.
Put-down	Let the elder know that you will listen in a nonjudgmental manner.

When you find yourself having a communication problem during an activity, ask yourself if any of these barriers exist.

SPECIAL SITUATIONS

During activity sessions, situations that merit special concern or consideration may occur. For any activity that requires the elder and leader to come into direct physical contact, the participants need to adhere to currently accepted practices for minimizing the chance of spreading infectious diseases.

Procedures to follow for exercise stress and falls are covered on pages 17 through 19. To prepare for these and other possible situations, be thoroughly familiar with the procedures specified by the sponsoring agency. Reviewing these procedures should be part of the initial training session and ongoing leader support meetings, as needed.

It is recommended that as persons are identified to receive the program, appropriate contacts in case of emergency are determined; this might be a relative, neighbor, visiting nurse, landlord. In addition, the sponsoring agency should have a telephone number and contact person available to the leader in special situations. In certain cases, it may be best to recommend that an activity session be held only during the operating hours of the agency so that a contact can be quickly made. The leader should write down this information and keep it in a convenient and accessible place. For example, the leader could record the information on an index card and carry it in a wallet, purse, or tote bag. Or this information could be kept in the elder's telephone book.

The emergency number 911, if available, should be called only if it is an obvious emergency. This and other numbers of people to be called in special situations should be readily available. The leader should recognize personal limitations in dealing with special situations and should not attempt to overstep them.

Another situation of concern occurs when the elder attempts to extend the session. Ending an activity is sometimes difficult, a situation that needs special emphasis. Perhaps the best way to avoid a difficult ending to a session is prevention. The following ideas are presented as ways to help control how the time is spent during a session.

(a) Closely follow the activity plan format, beginning with "What to do during this session."

(b) As the activities are explained, briefly summarize what will occur during the session, clarifying expectations and briefly reviewing the structure of the activity; state the time available for the session.

(c) As the ending time draws near, begin expressing enjoyment and appreciation and make references to the next session; perhaps verbally note the current time. For example, "This has been an enjoyable session and I appreciate your company and participation. It's three o'clock, however, and it's time for me to leave until our next meeting."

(d) Use nonverbal exit clues such as partly or completely rising from a chair, lessening eye contact, glancing at the clock or one's watch, shaking the elder's hand, etc.

If the session time consistently runs longer than desired, the following ideas may be of assistance:

(a) Plan to conduct a portion of "Doing Activities" only. Do not attempt to finish the entire activity in one session.

(b) Provide a cheerful but firm reminder regarding the desired length of time of the session; seek a mutual agreement on the desired time limit. For example, in a lighthearted manner, state, "We have not been doing too well on ending our sessions on time! It's important for me to keep to about one hour in length, and I think that's best for you, too. Don't you agree?" In some situations, this reminder might need to be given at the beginning of each session.

(c) Begin ending the session after 40 to 45 minutes by giving a verbal signal that the time is almost up. For example, "Mary, I have just noticed that we have about ten minutes left. Let's review what we've done today and what we'll cover during the next session."

(d) If the senior continues to discuss new topics, respond, "I can see you still have some things you'd like to talk about, yet we don't have time today. Let's see when our next session is."

(e) Plan the session before a regularly scheduled activity. For example, one senior living in a retirement center regularly ate supper with the other residents at 5:30 p.m. Thus, the leader scheduled the sessions for 4:00 p.m., assuring that it would end within 1½ hours.

The leader should demonstrate by words and actions the intention to leave. That is, when the leader says it's time to leave and stands to leave, he/she should then leave! The elder will better understand the time limits if the leader consistently leaves at the designated time. If the leader states an intention to leave and then stays for an additional length of time, the signals will be confusing and lead to a belief that the leader really does have more time available.

Ending the session at the designated time does not mean rejection. In fact, sticking to the time limits will prove of greater benefit for both. End the session on an upbeat, positive note, making reference to the next one. In time, the elder will understand and appreciate the time limit and will realize that the leader will come again at the next designated time.

CONFIDENTIALITY

At times during the program, the leader will see, hear, write, or read confidential information. Confidential information is any communication to, or observation by, the leader which is not clearly intended to be shared with another person. Exceptions could be another person who is directly involved in providing services to the elder or program coordinator.

The elder may determine or control the nature of the information he/she wishes to disclose. If the elder chooses not to answer questions that the leader feels are important to conducting a safe and successful session, the leader should then contact the program coordinator for assistance. The leader should not collect any personal information that is clearly not necessary for the program.

Examples of confidential information include

Information given in confidence by the elder in the course of receiving the program activities.

Information that is given in confidence by family, friends, neighbors, etc.

Any opinion, summary or instruction concerning the elder given by sponsoring agency personnel in the course of the program.

Personal information which, if told to others, could possibly be detrimental to the best interests of the elder.

REFERENCES AND RESOURCES

Austin, D. R. Therapeutic recreation, processes and techniques. New York: John Wiley and Sons, 1982.

Austin, D. R., & Powell, L. G. Resource guide: College instruction in recreation for individuals with handicapping conditions. Bloomington, IN: Indiana University, 1980.

Bullock, C. C., Wohl, R. E., Webeck, T. E., & Crawford, A. M. Leisure is for everyone. Resource and Training Manual, Curriculum in Recreation Administration. Chapel Hill, NC: University of North Carolina at Chapel Hill, 1982.

Des Moines Area Community College. Activity director workshop manual. Estherville, IA: Iowa Lakes Community College, 1983.

Hamill, C. M., & Oliver, R. C. Therapeutic activities for the handicapped elderly. Rockville, MD: Aspen Systems Corporation, 1980.

Kraus, R. Therapeutic recreation service: Principles and practices (3rd ed.). Philadelphia: Saunders College Publishing, 1981.

Moran, J. M. Leisure activities for the mature adult. Minneapolis, MN: Burgess Publishing, 1980.

O'Morrow, G. S. Therapeutic recreation, a helping profession (2nd ed.). Reston, VA: Reston Publishing, 1980.

Peterson, C. A., & Gunn, S. L. Therapeutic recreation program design (2nd ed.). Englewood Cliffs, NJ: Prentice-Hall, 1984.

Purtilo, R. The allied health professional and the patient. Philadelphia: W. B. Saunders, 1973.

Russell, R. V. Leadership in recreation. St. Louis: Times Mirror/Mosby College Publishing, 1986.

Shivers, J. S., & Fair, H. F. Special recreational services: Therapeutic and adapted. Philadelphia: Lea and Febiger, 1985.

Stein, T. A., & Sessoms, H. D. Recreation and special populations (2nd ed.). Boston: Holbrook Press, 1977.

U.S. Department of Health, Education, and Welfare. Activities coordinator's guide. HE22.208; L85. Washington, DC: U.S. Government Printing Office, 1978.

Wehman, P., & Schleien, S. Leisure programs for handicapped persons. Baltimore: University Park Press, 1981.

CHAPTER 4

Exercise Assessment

But let there be no scales to weight your unknown treasure;
And seek not the depths of your knowledge with staff or
sounding line.
For self is a sea boundless and measureless.

--Kahlil Gibran

Assessment is time devoted to the measurement or evaluation of a person's current, past, or perceived future status. This can occur in a formal situation such as a student completing an exam, or informally as when the family sits around the dinner table discussing whether the dog or cat is sick and needs a trip to the veterinarian. Administering and interpreting formal assessments, such as an electrocardiogram or an IQ test, require special training. Informal assessments can be done by everyone; however, it is difficult to compare the results with other information.

Before engaging in a series of planned physical activities, some time should be spent assessing a person's current condition. This is even more important when the person is very old and/or frail. Without assessing condition, a leader risks failure in meeting the intended results of the unit, and will not know how best to meet the needs of the elder. Interpreting the assessment results will help the leader to get acquainted in a very short time. As an example of how an assessment can help an activity succeed, two hypothetical situations are presented below.

In one instance, the leader assesses the elder's visual abilities during the first session by informally looking over the tests of physical functioning. The elder and leader are sitting next to one another on a couch, in good lighting, with the elder holding the exercise book. The leader reads the directions of the Wall Test and then asks if there are any questions. If the elder has no questions, the leader asks the elder if he or she would like to read the description of the Sit-and-Reach Test. If the description is read, more is learned about his/her ability to see and read print. If the elder declines, the leader continues to read.

In a second situation, the leader has not previously assessed the ability to read the print before attempting to complete the unit on arthritis, diabetes, and Parkinson's disease. During a session some printed index cards are placed on the table in front of the elder. The leader asks the elder to read information from the material. Embarrassment results because the elder can't read the print. Rejection of the activity occurs, and the elder does not want to continue. Restarting the session using a different approach isn't possible now that the elder is defensive.

In the first situation, the elder always had a way to gracefully decline reading aloud. Reading was an option and was led into slowly. In the second situation, the elder was thrust headfirst into a reading task. By the time it became obvious that the reading was impossible, the activity was in progress and came to an uncomfortable halt. There was no alternative, except to admit the task was impossible.

Another important reason for assessing a frail person is that areas of serious concern or deficiency may be found. The leader can then inform the program coordinator about the problem. The coordinator can follow up by contacting a social service program. The leader has then helped to bring services other than exercise or recreation into that person's life.

In conclusion, it is important to keep assessment in perspective. A person cannot be understood by marks on a score sheet. A complete understanding of a person cannot be expected to develop rapidly. A clear understanding of the elder, from a variety of perspectives, will evolve as a unit progresses. The formal assessments of physical functioning, presented in the next section, are at best only an approximation of the true picture. The assessment activities should be enjoyed for themselves, with laughter, discussion, and possibly, disagreement along the way.

ASSESSING PHYSICAL FUNCTIONING

In preparation for an exercise unit, and to establish baseline values of physical functioning, three tests are recommended. Shoulder flexibility can be assessed by the Wall Test, hip flexibility by the Modified Sit-and-Reach Test, and strength by the Chair Test. Record the results of these tests using the following Physical Functioning Assessment Record Sheet.

Physical Functioning Assessment Record Sheet

Test	Pre-test score		Post-test score	
	Elder	Leader	Elder	Leader
Wall Test (in inches) If score is 0, is face turned? (Yes,no)	____	____	____	____
Modified Sit-and-Reach (A,B,C,D,E)	____	____	____	____
Chair Test (A,B,C,D,E)	____	____	____	____

The Wall Test

Stand facing a bare section of a wall, and put one arm out in front until the fingers are touching the wall. Walk forward with small steps while sliding your fingers up the wall. If you get to the point where your arm is over your head and your face is against the wall, then turn your face away from your arm and place your cheek against the wall. In this position, you have 180 degrees of shoulder flexion, which is very good. Now notice how close your feet are to the wall and measure with a ruler from your toes to the wall. Repeat with your other arm.

The leader should always do the test first and record the results on the physical functioning assessment record sheet. The leader then helps the elder complete the test and record results. This test allows the pair to know if range-of-motion exercises are needed. Shoulder flexibility is used when reaching for objects on overhead shelves and when putting on blouses, shirts, sweaters, jackets, and coats.

The Modified Sit-and-Reach Test

This test measures lower back and hip flexibility. THIS TEST IS NOT RECOMMENDED FOR PERSONS WITH HIP REPLACEMENTS, as the test encourages maximal hip flexion (past the safe 90-degree range). To perform this test, sit in a firm unupholstered chair and place a similar chair in front of you. Put your feet up on this chair until your feet and calves are supported by one chair and your rump is in the other chair. Both chairs should have the same seat height. Stretch your arms out in front and try to slide your fingers down your shins. Score your best efforts as follows:

E = touched knees
D = touched shins
C = touched top of foot
B = touched toes when they pointed to ceiling
A = touched toes when they pointed forward

Never allow your knees to bend in this test. Slide your fingers only until you feel a stretch but not to the point of pain.

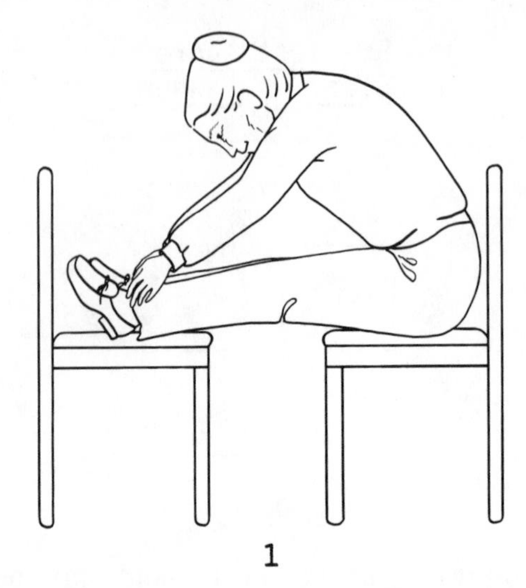

1

Lower back and hip flexibility are used when trying to pick up objects from the floor, when tying shoes and when trying to pull one's legs into a tight sitting situation like the front seat of a car or an auditorium seat. Poor flexibility in the lower back can cause lower back pain.

The Chair Test

The Chair Test is an assessment of lower body strength. THIS TEST ALSO REQUIRES SEVERE HIP FLEXION AND IS NOT RECOMMENDED FOR PERSONS WITH HIP REPLACEMENTS. Seat yourself in a hard chair that does not rock. Have your feet together and comfortably tucked back under the chair.

Level E

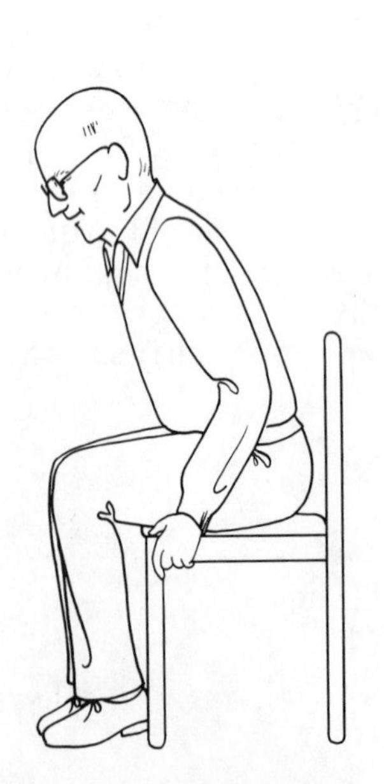

2

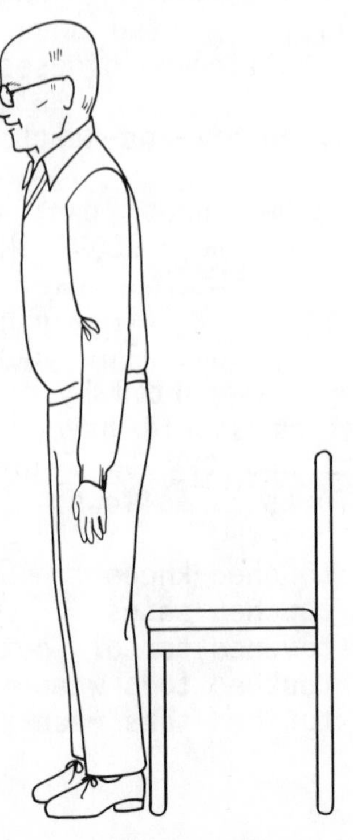

3

Place your hands on the front of the chair seat. Try to rise to a stand while using your hands to push. This is level E. If you complete it successfully, continue to the next level.

Level D

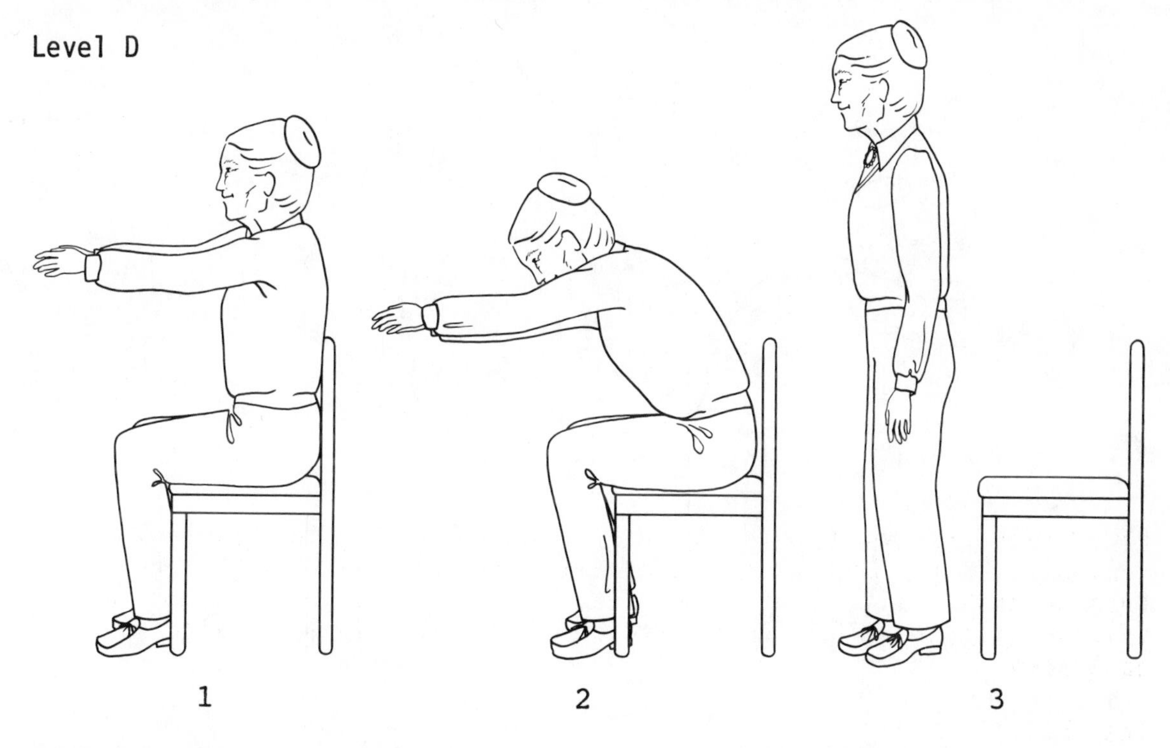

Begin level D by leaning back against the chair backrest. Hold your arms straight out in front of you. Now rock forward once and go into a stand. If you complete it successfully, continue to the next level.

Level C

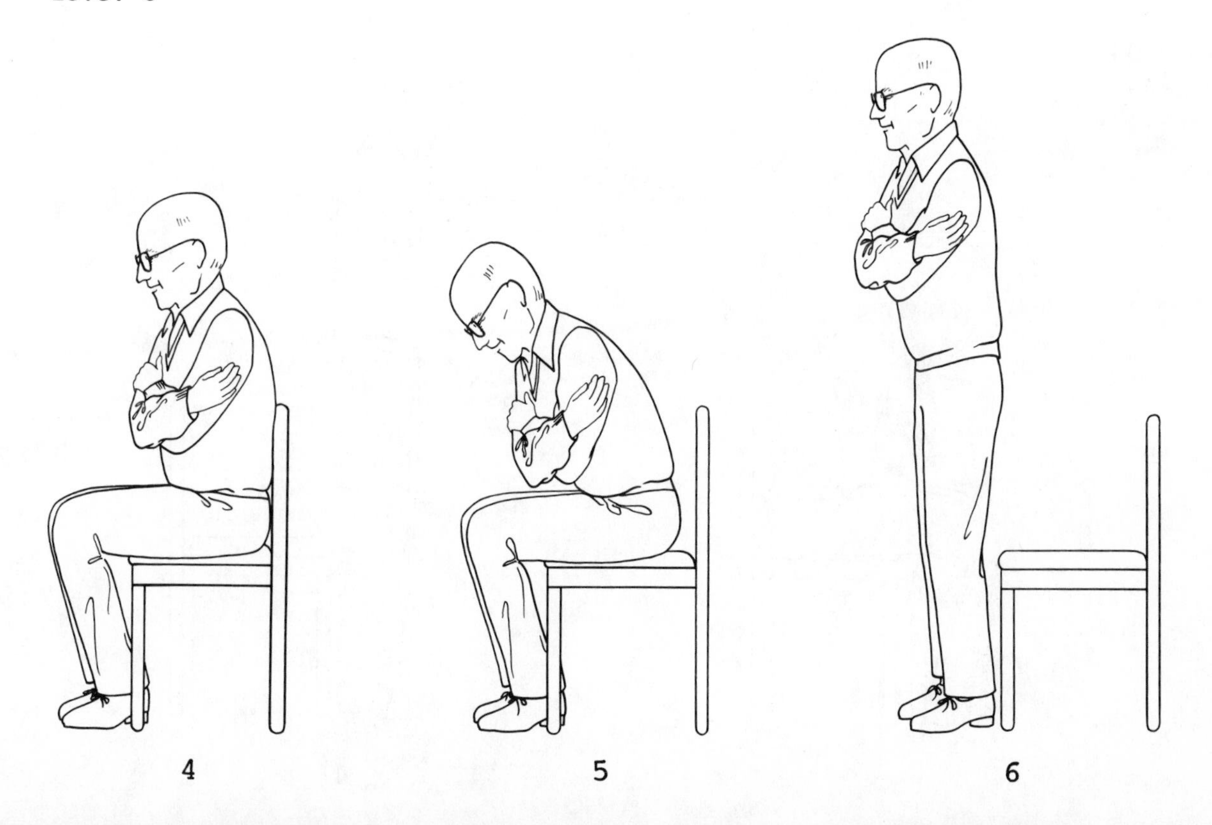

Begin level C by leaning back against the chair backrest and crossing your arms over your chest. Now rock forward once and go into a stand. If you complete it successfully, continue to the next level.

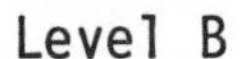

Level B

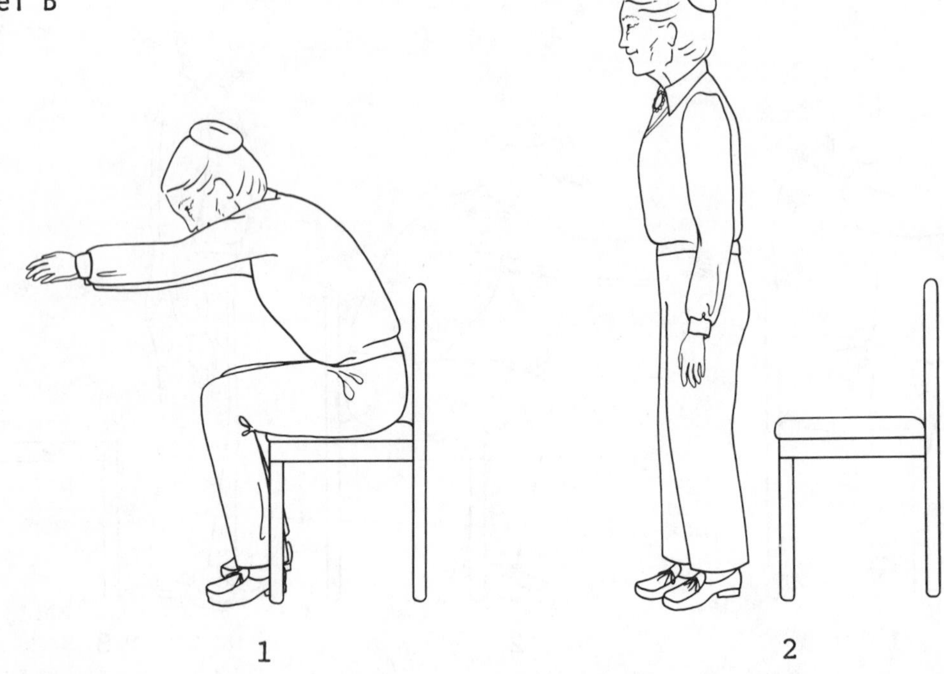

1 2

Begin level B from a stationary forward lean position with your arms straight out in front of you. Keeping this forward lean and forward reach, try to come to a stand. Do not count the trial if you moved or pumped your trunk to get started. If you completed it successfully, continue to the next level.

Level A

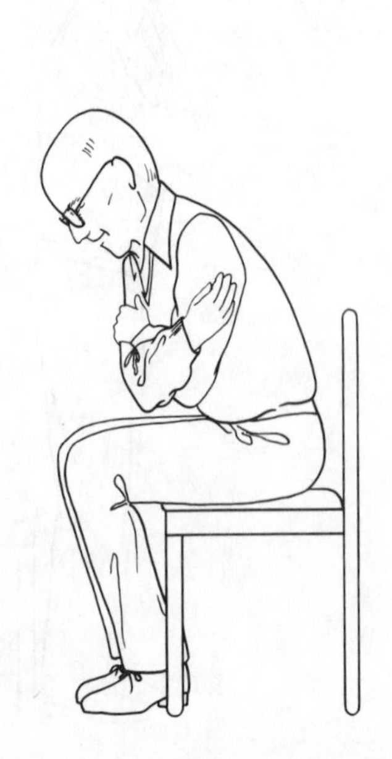

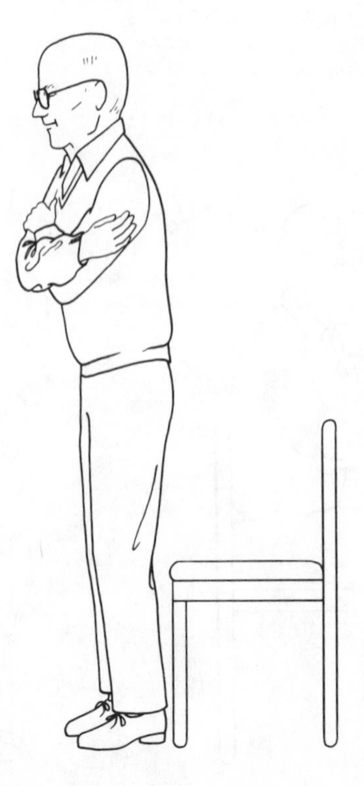

3 4

Begin level A from the stationary forward lean position with your arms crossed on your chest. Can you rise to a stand without moving your trunk first?

Lower body strength is needed to raise the body weight in stair climbing, rising from a chair, getting out of a bathtub, and rising from the floor.

ASSESSING OTHER PHYSICAL TASKS

The leader needs to know the elder's current condition in eyesight and hearing. These physical factors are used in every unit. Should a unit require modification, it is best if the leader can anticipate the changes needed.

Since declines in these physical tasks are sometimes an embarrassment to an older person, it is best to use informal techniques to identify current conditions. In addition, eyesight and hearing cannot be expected to change because of these program activities. The primary purpose for assessing these factors is to anticipate needed adaptations in activities.

It will be obvious during the first session if the elder has difficulty hearing. Other subtle clues are the presence of a telephone, record player, or radio. The leader can also simply ask if the elder enjoys listening to the radio.

The leader can purposely talk in different ways to see if the conversation is followed. For instance, turn away from the elder momentarily and say something. If the elder can still relate to what was said, hearing ability should be sufficient for the program activities without modification.

As mentioned earlier, sight and reading skills can be assessed by asking the elder to read the unit descriptions. A refusal to do so does not necessarily indicate a visual impairment; however, it does show a reluctance to join in activities that require reading.

REFERENCES AND RESOURCES

Gibran, K. The prophet. New York: Alfred A. Knopf, 1968.

PART II

Activities

CHAPTER 5

Special Features of the Program

STARTING A UNIT

Chapter 2, "Learning about Exercise," discussed physician approval as the first step in starting an exercise unit. Mailing or delivering the activity plans, illustrations, and/or exercise charts from Appendix B or Appendix C to the elder's doctor is the preferred process. The doctor can then write comments on the exercise descriptions or illustrations when omission or modification is needed.

While the doctor is evaluating the unit, it is possible to conduct a session using the activity plan for assessing physical functioning that follows. The results can be recorded and discussed at the close of the session. If physician approval is not received by the second session, the leader can offer the Making Exercise Equipment activity plan from Chapter 6, "Exercises for Strength." The items made during this session are useful in many exercises.

COMMUNITY RESOURCE REFERRAL

After nine or ten sessions have been completed, the leader and elder should be well acquainted. This will be the appropriate time to spend one session on networking the elder into exercise activities in the community. In some institutional settings such a transition may be impossible; however, delivered services can be encouraged for even the most severely restricted.

An activity plan to help the leader structure this session can be found on pages 49 through 52. Resources specific to each community must be identified by the leader or program coordinator prior to this session. This activity plan is usable with any unit.

ENDING A UNIT

The last session in a unit serves two purposes. First, the leader can follow up on the community resource referral session. It is important to verify that contacts were made and that the elder and program directors are communicating. The second purpose is to allow the elder a chance to reflect on the unit and repeat any favorite activities.

No activity plan is included for this session, as the direction and flow should come from the elder. After the leader finishes the greeting and opening chat, paying attention to immediate needs, it is appropriate to ask the elder, "Mary, of the activities that we have done together over the past 11 weeks, which would you like to repeat today?" The leader should be prepared for responses such as, "Oh! Why don't we just visit today?", or "I don't know, you decide." Such responses will be disappointing, as one of the goals of the program is to foster independence and control. It is recommended that the leader follow the "let's visit" suggestion with visiting, as this is a choice and decision expressed by the elder. In the case of the "don't know" response, the leader can try naming activities completed together, in the hope that the elder will select some.

In preparation for this session the leader needs to have <u>all</u> of the "things to take" items in the tote basket. The elder may wish to repeat any of the 11 previous sessions, including the tests of physical functioning.

ACTIVITY UNITS

The following units, Chapters 6 through 8, each contain activity plans for nine sessions. The Exercises for Strength unit is the most physically demanding unit, using extra resistance after the third session. Exercises for Arthritis, Diabetes, and Parkinson's Disease and Exercises for Special Purposes are both low-intensity units. Selection of these units will depend on the unique conditions the elder wishes to address.

Other activity units of a recreational nature can be found in the accompanying volume, <u>Recreation Activities for the Elderly</u>.

Appendix B includes illustrations and directions for the Exercises for Strength unit. Appendix C has illustrations and directions for the Exercises for Arthritis, Diabetes, and Parkinson's Disease unit. Both appendices use a bar code for each exercise. Numbers on the bar show which sessions use that exercise. Each activity plan also names the exercises to perform during that session. Numbers associated with the exercise help the reader locate the exercise in the proper appendix.

Each of the exercise units should begin with the session on assessment that follows.

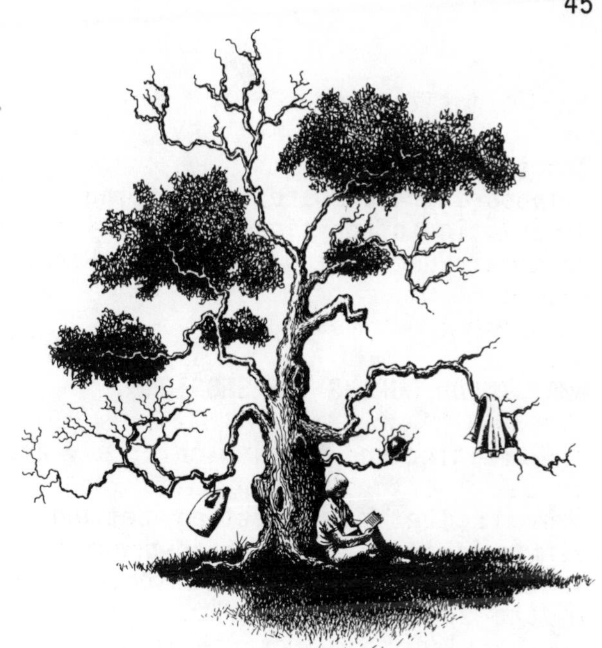

UNIT NAME: All Exercise Units

ACTIVITY PLAN 1: ASSESSING PHYSICAL FUNCTIONING

PURPOSE OF ACTIVITY: To learn the physical functioning levels of the elder and leader. To provide an opportunity for the elder and leader to get to know each other.

DESCRIPTION OF ACTIVITY: The elder and leader will complete the three tests of physical functioning described on pages 34 to 39.

BENEFITS OF ACTIVITY: This session provides some objective information about the elder and leader which can lead to conversations about personal physical weaknesses and needed areas of improvement. Information gained in this session will help the leader prepare for future sessions, and provides a baseline for measuring improvement.

BEFORE THE SESSION

Things to do

1. Phone the elder to schedule the session time. Make a short personal visit as an introduction if the elder seems troubled or skeptical about the program.

2. Photocopy the tests of physical functioning and the Physical Functioning Assessment Record Sheet from pages 34 to 39.

Things to take

Pencil
Clipboard or lapboard for writing
Description of physical functioning tests
Physical Functioning Assessment Record Sheet
Ruler

WHAT TO DO DURING THE SESSION

Greeting and opening chat; pay attention to immediate needs.

This is the first meeting between the elder and leader. It may be difficult to do a paper-and-pencil activity with the elder for a variety of physical or mental reasons. The leader must be ready to adapt, on the spot, to such situations. One of the most likely difficulties is the elder's reluctance to do any activity beyond talking. A second problem may result if the elder distrusts the paper-and-pencil approach with a stranger. For a variety of reasons the leader may need to talk about the elder's physical capabilities informally. It is very likely that a reluctance to do the tests of physical functioning is an indication that the elder is not ready for structured activity. In such cases the "Remembering the Past" unit from the Recreation Activities for the Elderly volume is recommended.

Explain the session's activities.

Do activities.

The leader demonstrates the Wall Test and scores his/her results. Next the leader assists the elder in trying the same test, and records the results.

The leader demonstrates the Sit-and-Reach Test and scores his/her results. Next the leader assists the elder in trying the same test, and records the results.

The leader demonstrates the Chair Test and scores his/her results. Next the leader assists the elder in trying the same test, and records the results.

Both persons can now look at the three exercise units, and choose one to do over the next 11 weeks.

Session wrap-up; enjoy a snack if desired.

As this is the first session, the elder probably will not have prepared a snack or even have realized that it is part of the program. The leader should have a snack to share with the elder at this time.

ENDING THE SESSION:

Talk about and confirm next session.

In preparation for the unit the leader needs to know if the elder has had a hip replacement and should ask for the name, address, and phone number of the elder's physician. Explain the importance of the physician's approval of the exercise program. If the elder does not want to involve the physician, it is best that another unit be selected. If the elder has not seen his/her physician in many years, the leader may suggest making an appointment and accompanying the elder on that trip. In such cases, be sure to take the exercise unit along to give to the physician.

AFTER THE SESSION:

Write up comments.

Make notes about observations made during the session regarding the elder's sight, hearing, and use of hands. Any limitations that might affect the elder's participation can be noted for adaptations in unit activities.

IDEAS FOR MODIFYING THE SESSION: No assessment should be given if the elder does not want to participate. The conversation approach mentioned in the "Greeting and opening chat" section of this activity plan is an important adaptation. The leader may also choose to do the Tests of Physical Functioning and let the elder watch. As the leader assesses his/her functioning, the elder may be drawn into the conversation and activity.

TIPS FOR SAFETY: Do not do the Chair Test or the Sit-and-Reach Test if the elder has had a hip replaced.

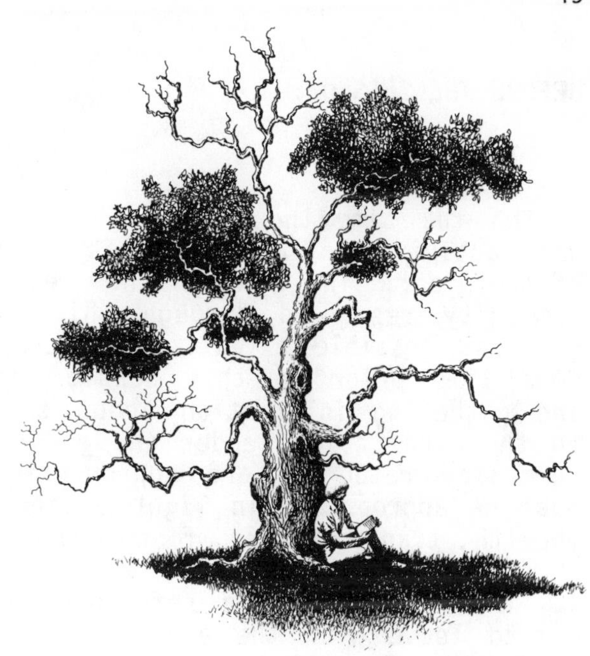

UNIT NAME: All Units

ACTIVITY PLAN 11: COMMUNITY RESOURCE REFERRAL

PURPOSE OF ACTIVITY: To present the elder with knowledge about various community resources through which interests developed during the course of any unit may be continued, and the needs for instrumental support can be met.

DESCRIPTION OF ACTIVITY: The leader will describe various community resources for seniors. Some resources should pertain to the topics of the units, others to the general well-being of the elder. With the help of the leader, the elder will:

1. Verbalize how he/she would like to pursue an interest in a unit topic.

2. Identify specific community resources he or she would like to contact.

3. Develop a specific plan for contacting these resources.

BENEFITS OF ACTIVITY: The leader identifies various community resources through which the elder can continue pursuing interests in the unit topic. Through this referral process the leader is helping the elder to discover ways to engage in this exercise activity without the help of the leader. This session helps to involve the elder in activities of the community to the greatest possible extent. Involvement in community activities is stressed, regardless of extent. This session also shows the elder that other services are available to help seniors meet nutritional, transportation, and health needs.

BEFORE THE SESSION:

Things to do

During the time the leader and elder have been participating in the unit activities, the leader has learned about the interests and needs of the elder. The leader is now ready to refer the elder to appropriate community resources through which interests can be pursued to the greatest possible extent. To accomplish this, the leader must spend some time prior to this session locating local community resources and gathering information about services and opportunities available to the elder. The leader and elder will determine which of the local community resources are appropriate to pursue. Community resources must be appropriate in light of the interests, needs, and limitations (health, transportation, finances) of the elder.

1. The leader makes a reference list of related community resources to leave with the elder. For example, an index card containing names of contact people and their phone numbers could be left by the telephone, tacked to a bulletin board, or inserted in a phone book. Listed below are examples of organizations, agencies, or personnel that may provide information to the leader.

   Park and recreation departments, districts, or commissions
   Senior centers
   YMCAs or YWCAs
   Churches and other service-oriented groups
   County extension offices
   Individuals from the community
   Merchants selling materials for various exercise needs
   Libraries--excellent sources for the names and locations of organizations and individuals and good resources in themselves
   Chambers of Commerce
   Yellow pages in the phone book

2. To learn about services designed to help seniors in institutions or in their homes, the leader should contact the Area Agency on Aging. Listed below are examples of services to help provide instrumental support to such persons.

   Home-delivered meals
   Home health care
   Homemaker service
   Transportation assistance
   Legal aid
   Handyman chore service

Things to take

Paper or index cards
Pencil
Resource materials (any pamphlets and brochures that are available)

WHAT TO DO DURING THE SESSION:

Greeting and opening chat; pay attention to any immediate needs.

Complete any unfinished business from previous session.

Explain the session's activities.

Do activities.

Discuss various community resources of interest to the elder by describing the type of service available from each resource and suggesting how this resource might be utilized. Assist the elder in selecting appropriate resources for future contact.

Once preferred resources have been selected, discuss how these might be contacted. On a piece of paper or index card write the following information:

1. Name of the agency and/or individual resource person.
2. Address and telephone number.
3. Type of service.
4. Various questions the elder would like to ask (such as questions about cost, transportation, mailing list, meeting time, and meeting place).

Discuss with the elder plans to contact these selected resources during the upcoming week(s). Determine the best day and time to make the initial contact; this day and time may be recorded on the piece of paper or index card containing the other information about the resource. Encourage the elder to write down important information received from the agency or individual resource person as a result of the contact. This information, also recorded on the piece of paper or index card, may be used for future reference and for discussion during the next session.

Session wrap-up; enjoy a snack if desired.

ENDING THE SESSION:

Share the basket.

Talk about and confirm next session.

Explain to the elder that in the next session, his/her progress in contacting the identified resources will be discussed.

Ask the elder if there is an activity related to the unit topic that could be a part of the next session. If no new activities come to mind, ask which activities from the previous sessions could be repeated during the next session.

AFTER THE SESSION:

Write up comments.

It is a good idea for the leader also to keep a written record of the specific resources the elder intends to contact. This list will aid the leader in following up the referral process in the next session.

IDEAS FOR MODIFYING THE SESSION: If the elder cannot read or write or does not appear motivated to follow through on referrals, the leader may offer to help make the contact. This decision is left to the best judgment of the leader. If the leader helps make these contacts, he/she should follow the procedure discussed below.

Assist in the process of contacting the agencies or individual resource person by dialing the phone and explaining that Mr. or Mrs. Jones is calling to inquire about the service. Then give the phone to the elder to make the actual inquiry.

It may be appropriate to ask the resource agency or person to make the initial contact with the elder. If so, the leader should be certain the elder has given permission for this contact to be made.

The leader is encouraged to display patience and understanding, as the elder may be very hesitant in responding to this session.

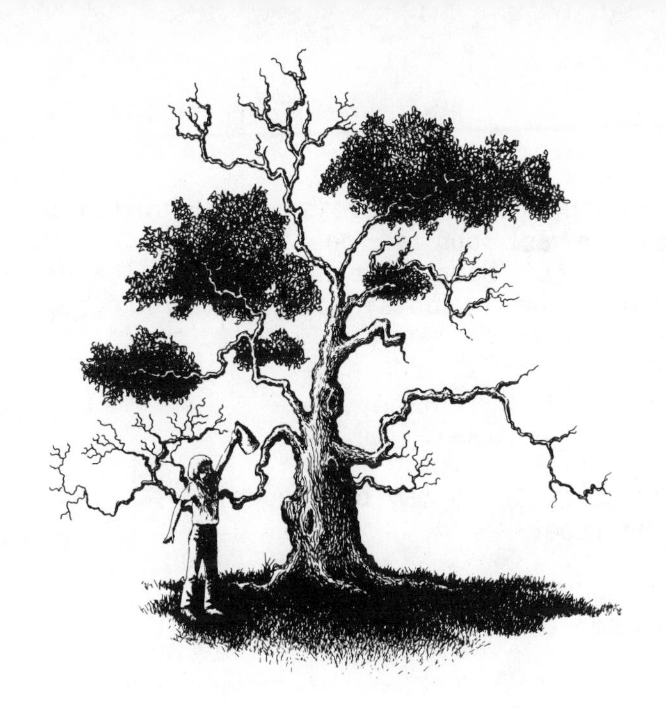

CHAPTER 6
Exercises for Strength

UNIT NAME: Exercises for Strength

(The first activity plan in all exercise units should be ASSESSING PHYSICAL FUNCTIONING. See pages 45 to 47.)

ACTIVITY PLAN 2: MAKING EXERCISE EQUIPMENT

PURPOSE OF ACTIVITY: To prepare the objects needed for strengthening muscles of the body and to demonstrate some of the exercises using extra weights.

DESCRIPTION OF ACTIVITY: The leader will assist the elder in making a plastic bottle hand weight, two tin can hand weights, two leg weights, and a rubber inner tube band. The leader will also perform some of the exercises using this equipment while the elder refers to the exercises illustrated in Appendix B.

BENEFITS OF ACTIVITY: This activity will allow the elder and leader to become further acquainted away from the structure required by the exercise patterns. Both can also make the equipment to match their individual strength capabilities. The elder will be introduced to the exercises and the illustrations in Appendix B. Areas of the body strengthened by each exercise can be discussed.

BEFORE THE SESSION

Things to make or do

The leader should clean four plastic bottles with handles. Detergent bottles are ideal. The leader should also procure two bicycle inner tubes. See the "doing activities" section of this activity plan for a description of how to find tubes and tube sizes. The program coordinator or leader must send a copy of the exercise unit including Appendix B to the elder's physician as soon as possible for review and approval. If the material has not been returned to the leader prior to this activity, another copy must be obtained from the program coordinator for use in the demonstration.

Things to take

Two plastic bottles
Filler for socks and bottles (as much as 10 lb may be needed)
Magic Marker or adhesive or masking tape
Two inner tubes
Scissors
A funnel to fill bottles; folded paper can often work as well
Two folding chairs if none are available
Four 1-lb cans of fruit or vegetables
Eight old socks
Appendix B with illustrations of the exercises

WHAT TO DO DURING THE SESSION:

Greeting and opening chat; pay attention to any immediate needs.

Ask the elder if there are any joints in his/her body that have been injured or do not have full range of motion. If there are some joints with problems, ask if there is pain when moving that joint. Explain that a copy of the exercise illustrations from Appendix B has been given to the elder's physician for specific approval of each exercise.

Complete any unfinished business from previous session.

Explain the session's activities.

Do activities.

1. Make plastic bottle hand weights

Take a plastic detergent or pancake syrup bottle that is clean, empty, and dry. Fill the bottle with dried peas, lentils, beans, rice, or any other granular material to give the bottle extra weight. The amount added to the bottle depends on how heavy you want it to be. No more than 1 lb is recommended for the elder and 2 to 3 lb for the leader. If you do not have a food scale at home, note the weight on the bag of food used. By keeping track of what portion of the bag you use, the weight in the bottle can be estimated. Using water to fill the bottles is a simple and easy way to get an exact measure of weight.

Using a 1-cup measure, put in 2 cups of water for 1 lb of weight. Although 1 lb seems light, it will provide a fair amount of resistance when held in the positions for exercise. Make a bottle for the elder and a bottle for the leader. Label the outside of the bottle with the user's name and the weight of the bottle. A Magic Marker can be used to mark directly on the bottles or ink pen can be used on masking or adhesive tape.

2. Make bicycle inner tube bands

Local bike shops are a good source for used inner tubes. Use the yellow pages to call businesses that service bicycles. Ask the dealer to save two inner tubes from flat tires. The size of the tube should be approximately 27" x 1¼" to 27" x 1½". This is important in order to give the correct amount of stretch and resistance. You will need two of these tubes, one for the elder and one for the leader. Bike shops usually give such tubes away, as they are unusable.

Once you have the tubes, cut the tube on both sides of the air nozzle and throw the nozzle away. Tie a knot in the free ends to re-form the loop. Next wash the tubes in soapy water.

3. Make can hand weights

Look in your cupboards for 1-lb cans of fruits or vegetables. The elder and leader will each need 2 cans of equal size and weight. These are ready to use immediately. It is not necessary to remove the labels.

4. Make leg weights

Fill each sock with about 1 lb beans or other granular material. Tie the open ends of 2 socks together. The result is a handy 2 lb leg weight as illustrated below. Each person will need two sock leg weights.

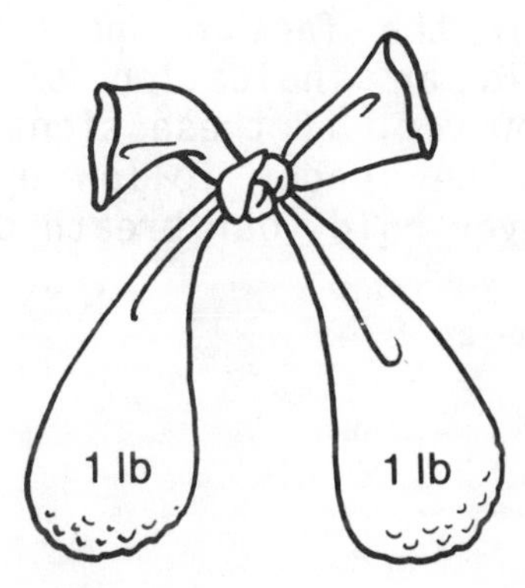

5. Demonstrate the exercises

The elder can sit next to the leader, allowing enough space for the leader to do the exercises, yet close enough so that both can see the illustration. The leader demonstrates the exercises, and the elder and leader refer to the "anatomy man" to find the area of the body strengthened in each exercise. These exercise and anatomy illustrations are located in Appendix B. If there is any confusion as to the exact movements in an exercise, a mark can be placed on the illustration for that exercise. During the next week the leader can refer to the written explanation of the exercises in the next three activity plans in this unit. If the illustrations from Appendix B are still with the physician, an extra copy must be obtained from the program coordinator to use during this demonstration.

Session wrap-up; enjoy a snack if desired.

ENDING THE SESSION:

Share the basket.

Talk about and confirm next session.

AFTER THE SESSION:

Write up comments.

IDEAS FOR MODIFYING THE ACTIVITY:

TIPS FOR SAFETY: Always demonstrate the exercises slowly. Explain to the elder that slower motions make the muscles work, whereas rapid motions use momentum to keep the body moving. Slower exercises will not put a strain on the cardiovascular system. Exercising to strengthen the heart is not the intent of this exercise program. Explain to the elder that if he/she ever notices difficulty in talking while exercising or flushing of the face or perspiration above the lip or on the forehead, this is an indication of a normal cardiovascular response to exercise. However, if these signs appear, the elder should stop exercising and let the leader follow up on how to continue the program safely. Also, never hold your breath during exercises.

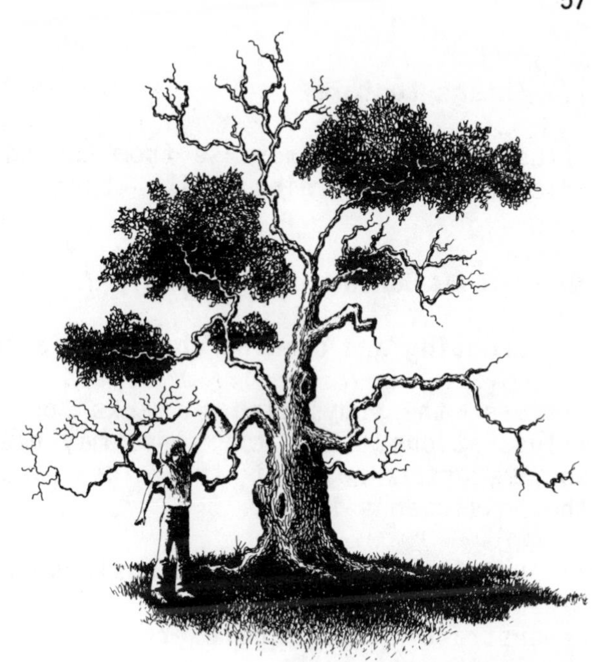

UNIT NAME: Exercises for Strength

ACTIVITY PLAN 3: LEARNING THE MOVES

PURPOSE OF ACTIVITY: To learn the proper positions for several exercises and complete three repetitions of each exercise without using extra weights.

DESCRIPTION OF ACTIVITY: The leader and the elder will exercise together from armless chairs. The leader will review the demonstration and explanation of the exercises to the elder. Three repetitions of each exercise are recommended.

BENEFITS OF ACTIVITY: This session will begin the progressive exercise program by working all of the major muscles of the body. The extra hand weights will not be used, and each exercise will be repeated only three times. This makes the exercises easy and gives the elder and leader a base to build on. Recording the completed exercises will be motivating to the elder.

BEFORE THE SESSION:

Things to make or do

The leader will prepare a means for marking on the exercise chart. This can be in the form of stick-on stars or symbols. Stickers can be purchased in quantity at bookstores or drugstores. The leader should follow up on any exercises that were marked as confusing during the demonstration in last week's session.

Things to take

Illustrations and exercise from Appendix B
Stickers for recording on the chart

WHAT TO DO DURING THE SESSION:

Greeting and opening chat; pay attention to any immediate needs.

Discuss the physician's marks on the exercise unit or appended illustrations. Some exercises may need to be omitted, and these should be discussed so that the elder and leader both clearly understand the physician's intent.

Complete any unfinished business from previous session.

Demonstrate all of the exercises that were marked as confusing during the last session.

Explain the session's activities.

Do activities.

Do three repetitions of each of the following exercises without using weights. Refer to Appendix B for illustrations and directions for these exercises. Numbers refer to the exercise numbers in the appendix for ease in location.

1. Toast your arms
2. Take a little drink
5. Swim the breast stroke
9. March a mile
12. Scissor your legs
24. Plié a little
26. Tippy toes
6. Climb a rope
13. Flutter kick

Session wrap-up; enjoy a snack if desired.

Begin recording the exercises on the record chart found in Appendix B. Discuss the importance of strengthening the muscle groups in these exercises. The listing below will help in this discussion:

1. "Swim the breast stroke" helps maintain strength and range of motion for putting on jackets and sweaters.

2. "March a mile" and "Plié a little" help strengthen thigh muscles for rising from a chair and climbing stairs.

3. "Scissor your legs" strengthens muscles of the hip joint, which help stabilize the hip during walking.

4. "Tippy toes" strengthens calf muscles for walking and climbing stairs.

ENDING THE SESSION:

Share the basket.

Talk about and confirm next session.

AFTER THE SESSION:

Write up comments.

IDEAS FOR MODIFYING THE ACTIVITY: If there is a joint with complications for either the elder or the leader, avoid the exercises using that joint.

TIPS FOR SAFETY: Always do the exercises slowly. Slower motions make the muscles work, whereas rapid motions use momentum to keep the body moving. Slower exercises will not put a strain on the cardiovascular system. Exercising to strengthen the heart is not the intent of this program. If you should notice difficulty in talking while exercising or flushing of the face or perspiration above the lip or on the forehead, this is an indication of a normal cardiovascular response to exercise. However, if you see these signs you should stop exercising and consult a physician to see if these exercises are too strenuous for your heart.

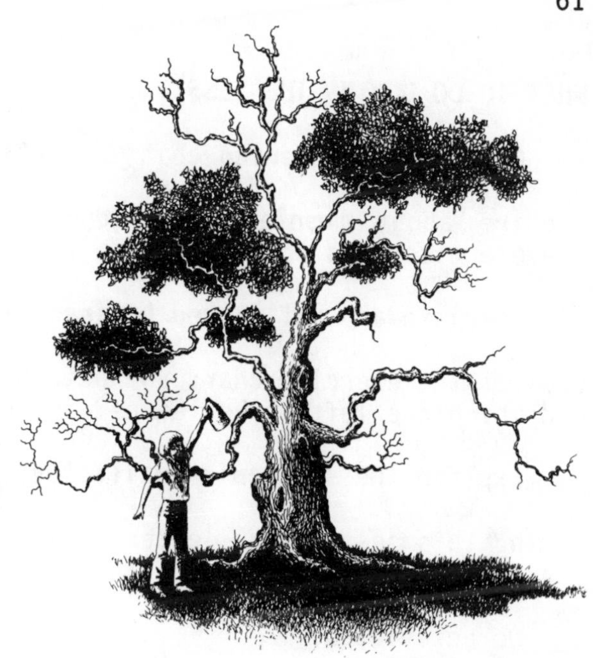

UNIT NAME: Exercises for Strength

ACTIVITY PLAN 4: MORE NEW MOVES

PURPOSE OF ACTIVITY: To continue learning the exercises for this unit.

DESCRIPTION OF ACTIVITY: The leader will lead the elder through the exercises in today's session. Repetitions still remain at three with no extra weights. Recording today's exercises on the chart will finish this session.

BENEFITS OF ACTIVITY: This session continues the learning of the exercises, excluding those using the inner tube. The resistance in these exercises is still low, as no external weights are used and repetitions are few. The elder and leader also locate the muscles strengthened in each exercise illustrated in Appendix B.

BEFORE THE SESSION:

Things to make or do

Things to take

Exercise chart
Stickers to mark progress
Exercise illustrations from Appendix B

WHAT TO DO DURING THE SESSION:

Greeting and opening chat; pay attention to any immediate needs.

Inquire about muscle or joint soreness to see if the intensity of the exercises was appropriate in the last session.

Complete any unfinished business from previous session.

Look at the exercise chart and note how many exercises have been learned and which are left to be learned in the next two sessions.

Explain the session's activities.

During this session the leader will lead the elder through the remaining exercises except those using the inner tubes.

Do activities.

Do three repetitions of each of the following exercises. The numbers refer to the location of the exercise in Appendix B.

7. Take off your hat
10. Kick the football
25. Hot seat
8. Walk a tightrope
11. Raise your toes
27. Tighten your tummy (**warning**: try one leg at a time at first)
28. Stand up and shout
4. Sitting jacks
3. Swing a garden gate

Session wrap-up; enjoy a snack if desired.

During this time, record on the chart the exercises done in this session. Also look at the "anatomy man" drawings in Appendix B for each of the exercises learned in the unit to better understand what body parts are strengthened by the 18 exercises learned thus far. The leader can demonstrate the exercise while the elder locates the muscles on the diagrams.

ENDING THE SESSION:

Share the basket.

Talk about and confirm next session.

AFTER THE SESSION:

Write up comments.

IDEAS FOR MODIFYING THE ACTIVITY: If the elder has been able to learn and remember the exercises easily, the leader may wish to see how many of the exercises the elder can remember by name. The leader gives the name of the exercise, and the elder demonstrates one repetition.

TIPS FOR SAFETY: Always do the exercises slowly. Slower motions make the muscles work, whereas rapid motions use momentum to keep the body moving. Slower exercises will not put a strain on the cardiovascular system. Exercising to strengthen the heart is not the intent of this program. If you should notice difficulty in talking while exercising or flushing of the face or perspiration above the lip or on the forehead, this is an indication of a normal cardiovascular response to exercise. However, if you see these signs you should stop exercising and consult a physician to see if these exercises are too strenuous for your heart.

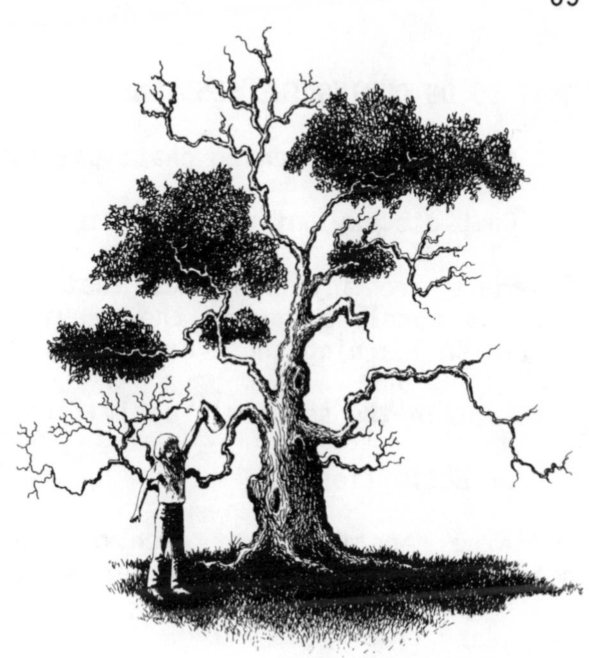

UNIT NAME: Exercises for Strength

ACTIVITY PLAN 5: INNER TUBE EXERCISES

PURPOSE OF ACTIVITY: To finish learning the exercises and to strengthen the muscles worked in this session.

DESCRIPTION OF ACTIVITY: The leader and the elder will exercise together from armless chairs. The leader will help demonstrate and explain the exercises to the elder. Three repetitions of each exercise are recommended.

BENEFITS OF ACTIVITY: This session will give a sense of accomplishment to the elder and leader, as they will have completed all of the exercises in the unit.

BEFORE THE SESSION:

Things to make or do

The leader should practice the exercises for today's session, as the use of the tubes may seem confusing at first.

Things to take

Exercise illustrations from Appendix B
Exercise chart
Inner tubes
Stickers for recording exercises

WHAT TO DO DURING THE SESSION:

Greeting and opening chat; pay attention to any immediate needs.

Complete any unfinished business from previous session.

If there are any exercises that the elder and leader have not been able to complete during the previous session, they may use this time to finish learning those exercises.

Explain the session's activities.

Do activities.

Do three repetitions of each of the following exercises. The numbers refer to the location of the exercise in Appendix B.

14. Bear trap
20. Pull on your sweater
16. Grandfather clock
21. Row-row-row your boat
17. Spread your legs
22. Stretch and yawn
19. Shoot the arrow
18. Brake your car
23. Lift the barbell

Session wrap-up; enjoy a snack if desired.

During this time record on the chart the exercises done in this session.

ENDING THE SESSION:

Share the basket.

Talk about and confirm next session.

AFTER THE SESSION:

Write up comments.

IDEAS FOR MODIFYING THE ACTIVITY: It may be too difficult for the elder to get the tube in position for the "Bear trap," "Mule kick," and "Grandfather clock" exercises. The leader can position the tube for the elder.

TIPS FOR SAFETY: Always do the exercises slowly. Slower motions make the muscles work, whereas rapid motions use momentum to keep the body moving. Slower exercises will not put a strain on the cardiovascular system. Exercising to strengthen the heart is not the intent of this program. If you should notice difficulty in talking while exercising or flushing of the face or perspiration above the lip or on the forehead, this is an indication of a normal cardiovascular response to exercise. However, if you see these signs, you should stop exercising and consult a physician to see if these exercises are too strenuous for your heart.

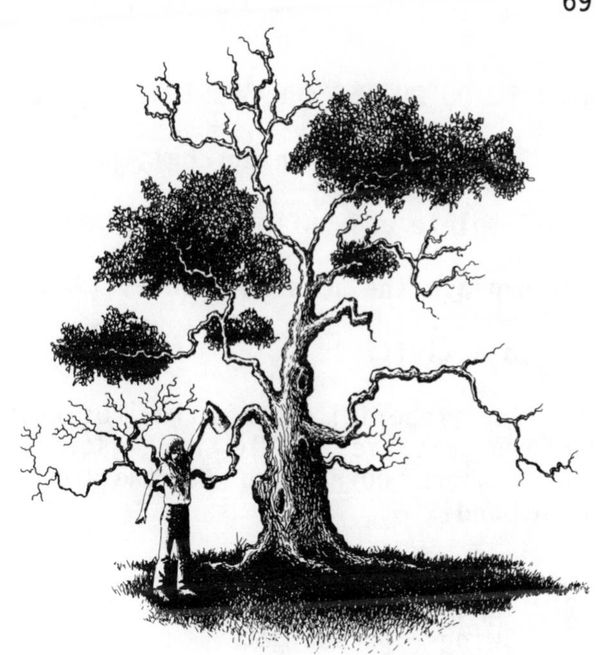

UNIT NAME: Exercises for Strength

ACTIVITY PLAN 6: ADDING WEIGHT

PURPOSE OF ACTIVITY: To add external weights to some of the exercises learned in this unit.

DESCRIPTION OF ACTIVITY: The leader and the elder will exercise together from armless chairs. The leader will help demonstrate and explain the exercises to the elder. The elder and leader will learn to use leg weights, cans, and weighted bottles. Five repetitions of each exercise are recommended.

BENEFITS OF ACTIVITY: This session builds on the already existing exercise program, giving the elder and the leader progressive resistance for building strength. This session also continues to use the exercise equipment made during the second session.

BEFORE THE SESSION:

Things to make or do

Things to take

Exercise illustrations in Appendix B
Exercise chart and stickers
Sock weights
Bottle weights
Can weights

WHAT TO DO DURING THE SESSION:

Greeting and opening chat; pay attention to any immediate needs.

Complete any unfinished business from previous session.

Explain the session's activities.

Do activities.

Do five repetitions of the following exercises holding a 1-lb can or the plastic bottle as described in the exercise descriptions. The numbers correspond to the location of the exercise illustration in Appendix B.

1. Toast your arms
2. Take a little drink
3. Swing a garden gate
4. Sitting jacks

9. March a mile
11. Raise your toes
12. Scissor your legs
13. Flutter kick

Session wrap-up; enjoy a snack if desired.

During this time record on the chart the exercises done in this session.

ENDING THE SESSION:

Share the basket.

Talk about and confirm next session.

AFTER THE SESSION:

Write up comments.

IDEAS FOR MODIFYING THE ACTIVITY: Since this is the fourth session, extra weight is used in each exercise. The elder may not be ready to increase at this rate. Modifications would include choosing only seven of the exercises to perform today. It may be necessary to modify the order of exercises. The first four exercises use upper body muscles and the last four exercises use lower body muscles. Perhaps the elder would prefer to alternate an upper body exercise with a lower body exercise. By now the elder and leader know the exercises well enough to be able to arrange the order to their preference.

TIPS FOR SAFETY: Always do the exercises slowly. Slower motions make the muscles work, whereas rapid motions use momentum to keep the body moving. Slower exercises will not put a strain on the cardiovascular system. Exercising to strengthen the heart is not the intent of this program. If you should notice difficulty in talking while exercising or flushing of the face or perspiration above the lip or on the forehead, this is an indication of a normal cardiovascular response to exercise. However, if you see these signs, you should stop exercising and consult a physician to see if these exercises are too strenuous for your heart.

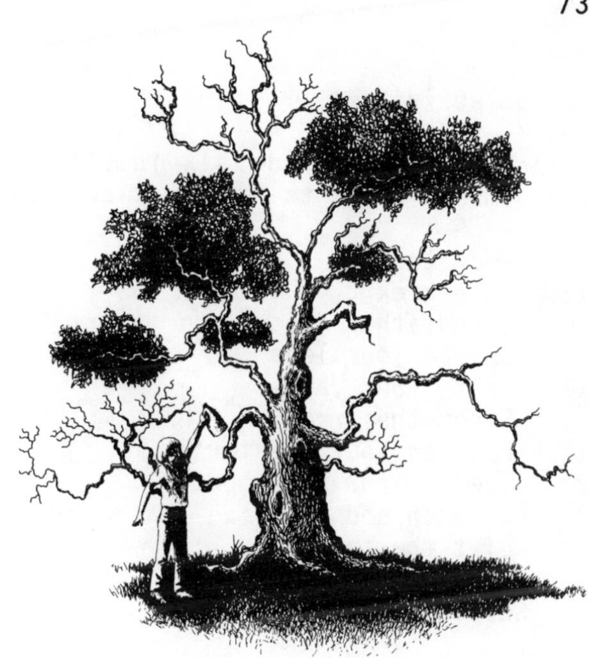

UNIT NAME: Exercises for Strength

ACTIVITY PLAN 7: STRETCHING TUBES

PURPOSE OF ACTIVITY: To continue strength exercises with inner tubes, adding additional repetitions to each exercise.

DESCRIPTION OF ACTIVITY: The leader and elder will exercise together from armless chairs using inner tubes for arms and legs.

BENEFITS OF ACTIVITY: This session repeats exercises learned in the unit with additional repetitions to build strength.

BEFORE THE SESSION:

Things to do

Things to take

Exercise illustrations and chart from Appendix B
Inner tubes
Stickers for recording on chart

WHAT TO DO DURING THE SESSION:

Greeting and opening chat; pay attention to any immediate needs.

Complete any unfinished business from previous session.

Explain the session's activities.

Do activities.

Using inner tubes, do six repetitions of each exercise as described. The numbers refer to the location of the exercise in Appendix B.

14. Bear trap
15. Mule kick
16. Grandfather clock
17. Spread your legs
18. Brake your car
19. Shoot the arrow
20. Pull on your sweater
21. Row-row-row your boat
22. Stretch and yawn
23. Lift the barbell

Session wrap-up; enjoy a snack if desired.

During this time record progress on the exercise chart.

ENDING THE SESSION:

Share the basket.

Talk about and confirm next session.

AFTER THE SESSION:

Write up comments.

IDEAS FOR MODIFYING THE ACTIVITY: Decrease the number of exercises or repetitions if necessary.

TIPS FOR SAFETY: Always do the exercises slowly. Slower motions make the muscles work, whereas rapid motions use momentum to keep the body moving. Slower exercises will not put a strain on the cardiovascular system. Exercising to strengthen the heart is not the intent of this program. If you should notice difficulty in talking while exercising or flushing of the face or perspiration above the lip or on the forehead, this is an indication of a normal cardiovascular response to exercise. However, if you see these signs, you should stop exercising and consult a physician to see if these exercises are too strenuous for your heart.

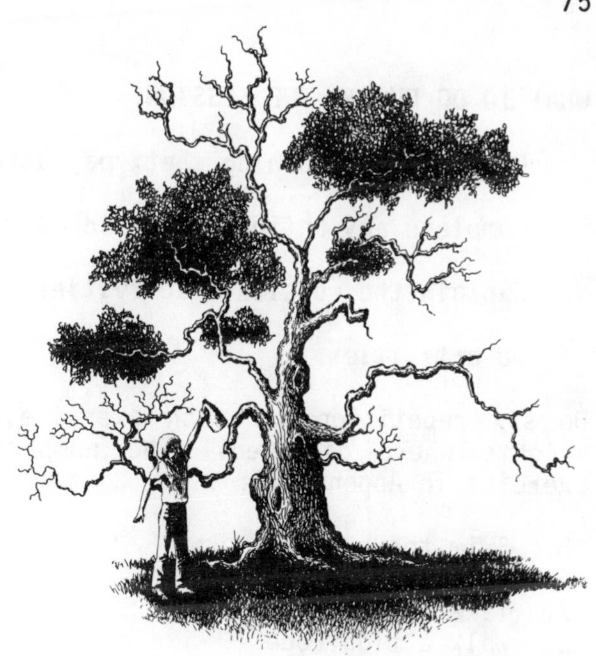

UNIT NAME: Exercises for Strength

ACTIVITY PLAN 8: TWICE THROUGH

PURPOSE OF ACTIVITY: To complete a second run through of all the exercises, using additional weights in the hands and one additional repetition.

DESCRIPTION OF ACTIVITY: The leader and elder will exercise together from an armless chair, using cans and bottles for hand weights.

BENEFITS OF ACTIVITY: This session is an important step in the unit progression. After this session is finished, the elder and leader will have completed every exercise twice with additional weight or repetitions the second time. After this session the elder will be encouraged to exercise on his/her own during the week.

BEFORE THE SESSION:

Things to make or do

Things to take

Exercise illustrations and chart from Appendix B
Exercise stickers
1-lb cans
Inner tubes
Sock weights
Plastic bottles
Wall calendar (optional)

WHAT TO DO DURING THE SESSION:

Greeting and opening chat; pay attention to any immediate needs.

Complete any unfinished business from previous session.

Explain the session's activities.

Do activities.

Do six repetitions of each exercise, using cans and bottles for hand weights where directed. The numbers refer to the location of the exercise in Appendix B.

5. Swim the breaststroke
6. Climb a rope
7. Take off your hat
8. Walk a tightrope
24. Plié a little
25. Hot seat
26. Tippy toes
27. Tighten your tummy (**warning:** Use one leg at a time if you are weak)
28. Stand up and shout
15. Mule kick
17. Spread your legs
10. Kick the football

Session wrap-up; enjoy a snack if desired.

During this time record progress on the exercise chart. Notice that all exercises have been done twice and that the second time through was with extra resistance.

ENDING THE SESSION:

Share the basket.

Talk about and confirm next session.

During the week before the next session the elder may want to do some of the exercises on his/her own time. To make this possible, the leader should leave the following for the elder.

Exercise illustrations from Appendix B
Cans
One inner tube
Socks
Two plastic bottles

Only one day of additional exercise is recommended and only ten exercises with six repetitions each.

AFTER THE SESSION:

Write up comments.

IDEAS FOR MODIFYING THE ACTIVITY: The most beneficial modification would be to reward this second time through the total package beyond the usual stickers. One suggestion is to give the elder a wall calendar with the session days crossed off on the calendar, plus a big star for today's session. Wall calendars are often free from businesses. The elder can use the calendar to mark an extra workout during the week.

TIPS FOR SAFETY: Always do the exercises slowly. Slower motions make the muscles work, whereas rapid motions use momentum to keep the body moving. Slower exercises will not put a strain on the cardiovascular system. Exercising to strengthen the heart is not the intent of this program. If you should notice difficulty in talking while exercising or flushing of the face or perspiration above the lip or on the forehead, this is an indication of a normal cardiovascular response to exercise. However, if you see these signs, you should stop exercising and consult a physician to see if these exercises are too strenuous for the heart.

Emphasize that the elder not overexercise during the week. The strength unit is carefully planned to increase the work done by each muscle group. If there are exercises using the standing posture or difficult inner tube positions, the elder may want to avoid these exercises during the week when the leader is not there to assist.

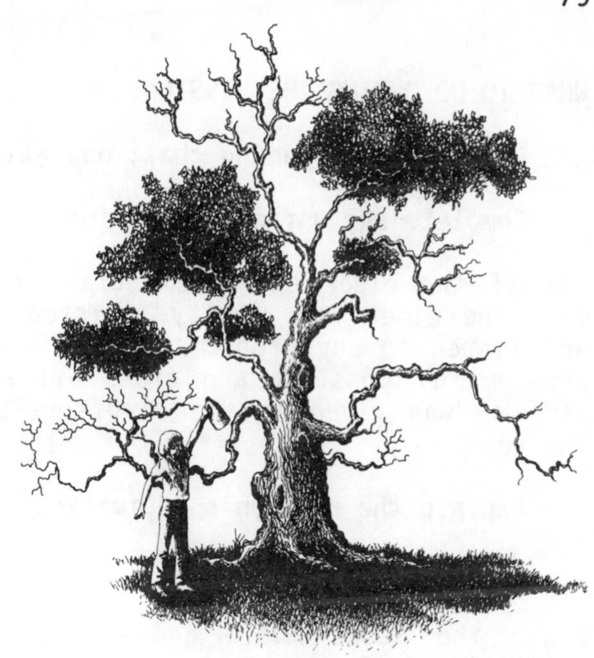

UNIT NAME: Exercises for Strength

ACTIVITY PLAN 9: SWINGING ALONG

PURPOSE OF ACTIVITY: To begin the third run-through of the exercises, adding more repetitions and increasing the number of exercises. To add the joy of music to the exercise environment.

DESCRIPTION OF ACTIVITY: The leader and elder will complete half of the prescribed exercises with six repetitions per exercise and with background music.

BENEFITS OF ACTIVITY: The intensity of this session is one of the highest of the unit. The strength gains should be noticeable to both the elder and leader as a reward for their continued effort. Music also adds variety to this session, as the exercises are becoming so familiar that the elder may be bored. This session also begins to transfer the leading of the exercises to the elder.

BEFORE THE ACTIVITY:

Things to make or do

Things to take

Inner tube
Plastic bottle
Cans
Socks
Stickers for the exercise chart
Exercise illustrations and chart from Appendix B
Cassette recorder and taped music

WHAT TO DO DURING THE SESSION:

Greeting and opening chat; pay attention to any immediate needs.

Complete any unfinished business from previous session.

Ask if the elder exercised during the week. If not, don't press or make the elder feel guilty. Listen to the reasons for not exercising and listen to any problems encountered while exercising. Help clarify problems if possible and cross off an extra day on the wall calendar (if one was given in the last session) for the extra exercise during the week.

Explain the session's activities.

Do activities.

Begin the taped music and use it for background while doing six repetitions of the following exercises. The numbers refer to the location of the exercise in Appendix B.

1. Toast your arms
2. Take a little drink
3. Swing a garden gate
4. Sitting jacks
9. March a mile
10. Kick the football
11. Raise your toes
12. Scissor your lets
13. Flutter kick
20. Pull on your sweater
21. Row-row-row your boat
22. Stretch and yawn
23. Lift the barbell
17. Spread your legs

Session wrap-up; enjoy a snack if desired.

During this time record on the exercise chart today's exercises.

ENDING THE SESSION:

Share the basket.

Talk about and confirm next session.

During the week before the next session the elder may want to do some of the exercises on his/her own time. To make this possible the leader should again leave the following for the elder.

Exercise illustrations from Appendix B
Cans
One inner tube
Socks
Plastic bottle

Only one day of additional exercise is recommended and only 10 exercises with 6 repetitions per exercise.

AFTER THE SESSION:

Write up comments.

IDEAS FOR MODIFYING THE ACTIVITY: The leader and elder may want to match the repetitions of the exercise to the first beat of each measure of the music. Care should be taken not to increase the rate, losing the effect of the weights or causing an increase in heart rate.

TIPS FOR SAFETY: Always do the exercises slowly. Slower motions make the muscles work, whereas rapid motions use momentum to keep the body moving. Slower exercises will not put a strain on the cardiovascular system. Exercising to strengthen the heart is not the intent of this program. If you should notice difficulty in talking while exercising or flushing of the face or perspiration above the lip or on the forehead, this is an indication of a normal cardiovascular response to exercise. However, if you see these signs, you should stop exercising and consult a physician to see if these exercises are too strenuous for your heart.

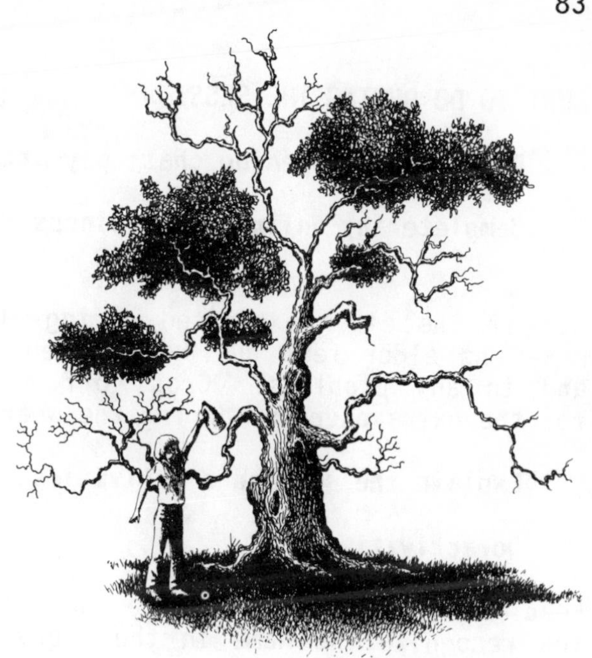

UNIT NAME: Exercises for Strength

ACTIVITY PLAN 10: AN EXERCISE STORY

PURPOSE OF ACTIVITY: To complete the third run-through of the exercise package and to add a novel approach in the form of a story to accompany the exercises.

DESCRIPTION OF ACTIVITY: The leader and elder will complete the fourteen remaining exercises listed in this unit while reading a story including the names of exercises.

BENEFITS OF ACTIVITY: Like the last session, the intensity of this session is one of the highest of the unit. The strength gains should be noticeable to both the elder and leader as a reward for their continued effort. The story also adds variety to this session.

BEFORE THE SESSION:

Things to make or do

Things to take

Inner tube
Plastic bottle
Cans
Socks
Stickers for the exercise chart
Exercise illustrations and chart from Appendix B

WHAT TO DO DURING THE SESSION:

Greeting and opening chat; pay attention to any immediate needs.

Complete any unfinished business from previous session.

Ask if the elder exercised during the week. If not, don't press or make the elder feel guilty. Listen to the reasons for not exercising and to any problems. Cross off an extra day on the wall calendar for the extra exercise during the week.

Explain the session's activities.

Do activities.

Read the following narrative and stop to do the exercises whenever you recognize the name in the story text. If you catch them all you will have done 14 exercises with 6 repetitions each.

While searching for firewood in the forest, two young boys found a bear trap. Deciding to carry the trap home with them, one of the boys took off his hat and used it like a purse to carry the trap. As they walked, they came upon a creek. One boy chose to swim the breast stroke across, while the boy with the trap spotted a fallen tree which he walked as a tightrope. Once on the other bank John, with the trap, said to Bill, his swimming friend, "Spread your legs as you kick and tighten your tummy as you stroke." As Bill emerged on the bank, John continued, "Pull on your sweater or you will freeze." As Bill crawled to the top of the bank he felt as if he had to stand up and shout: "I feel like I just received a big mule kick. Oh! It is cold." Bill did everything to get warm. He stood on his tippy toes, he plićd a little, and he ran in circles. Nothing helped, and both John and Bill became fearful. It was a brisk October day and they were miles from home. Bill had been foolish, but now it was too late to change the course of events. They knew they had to get home quickly to save Bill's life.

First, they decided to bury the trap so they could run to the car. The exercise would help keep Bill warm, and they could return to get the trap tomorrow. John used the trap to quickly dig a hole and then dropped the trap in the hole and covered it with loose dirt and a large rock to mark the spot. John crossed the creek quickly on the fallen tree; however, Bill was shaking so hard he could not balance. Spotting a vine on his side of the bank, John threw the end of the vine to Bill. "Climb a rope and swing across, Bill. I will catch you." Once Bill was in his arms, John held him close to warm his hands and body. Then they started running to the car.

When they reached the car, both boys were panting and Bill's face was aglow with the warm blood circulating rapidly from the run. John drove the 8 miles home in record time. He swung the car in the driveway so fast that Bill reacted by saying, "John, brake your car." John laughed as the car came to a halt. He knew Bill was home safe and he felt a relief rushing over his body. He too was feeling a chill as the sweat in his clothes from the run began to cool. In the house they both sat on the floor near the heating vent as the grandfather clock struck 5 p.m. "Can you believe we were only out there for 30 minutes, Bill?" John said jokingly. Bill replied, "It seemed like a lifetime once the air hit me on the creek bank." Then Bill and John jumped up with a yell. The vent had made quite a hot seat.

Session wrap-up; enjoy a snack if desired.

During this time record on the exercise chart for today's exercises.

ENDING THE SESSION:

Share the basket.

Talk about and confirm next session.

During the week before the next session the elder may want to do some of the exercises on his/her own time. To make this possible the leader should leave the following for the elder.

Exercise illustrations and record chart from Appendix B
Cans
One inner tube
Socks
Plastic bottle

Only two days of exercise are recommended, with ten exercises at six repetitions each.

AFTER THE SESSION:

Write up comments.

TIPS FOR SAFETY: Always do the exercises slowly. Slower motions make the muscles work, whereas rapid motions use momentum to keep the body moving. Slower exercises will not put a strain on the cardiovascular system. Exercising to strengthen the heart is not the intent of this program. If you should notice difficulty in talking while exercising or flushing of the face or perspiration above the lip or on the forehead, this is an indication of a normal cardiovascular response to exercise. However, if you see these signs, you should stop exercising and consult a physician to see if these exercises are too strenuous for your heart.

Emphasize that the elder not overexercise during the week. The strength unit is carefully planned to increase the work done by each muscle group.

REFERENCES AND RESOURCES

Chrisman, D. C. Body recall: A program of physical fitness for the adult. Berea, KY: Berea College Press, 1980.

Corbin, D. E., & Metal-Corbin, J. Reach for it! A handbook of exercise and dance activities for older adults. Dubuque, IA: Eddie Bowers Publishing, 1983.

Smith, E. Aging and exercise. Madison, WI: University of Wisconsin, 1978.

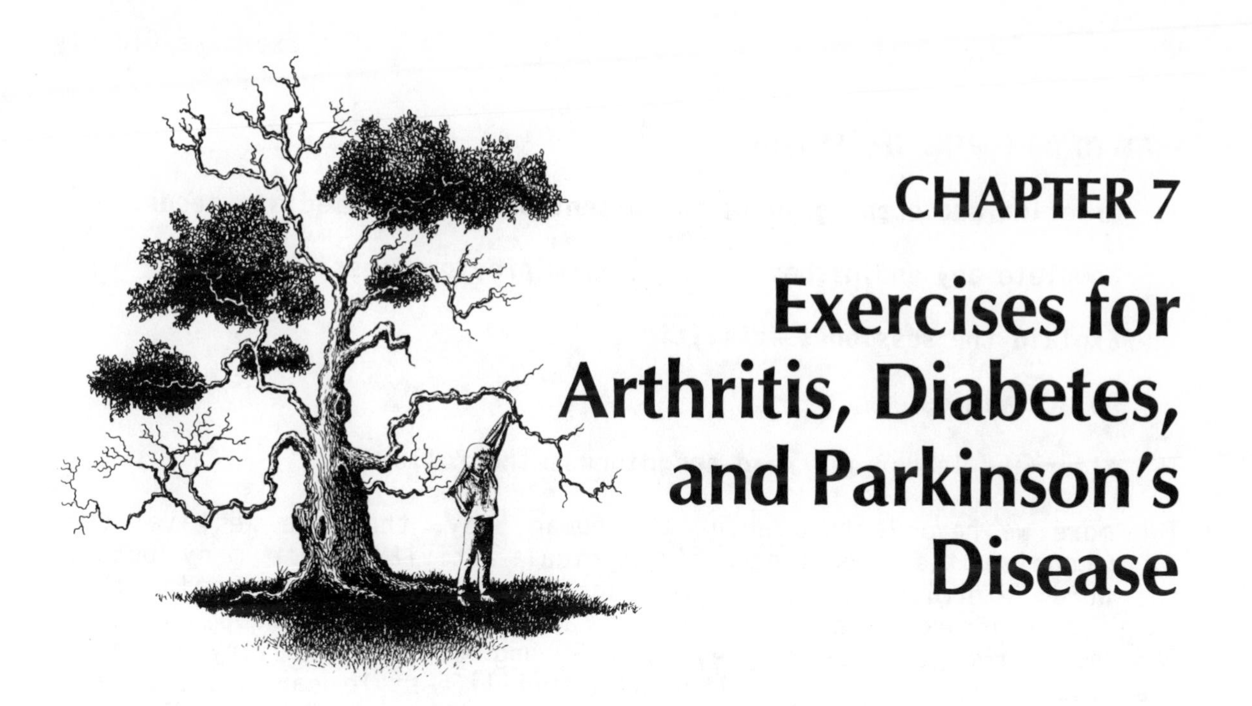

CHAPTER 7

Exercises for Arthritis, Diabetes, and Parkinson's Disease

UNIT NAME: Exercises for Arthritis, Diabetes, and Parkinsons's Disease

(The first activity plan in all exercise units should be ASSESSING PHYSICAL FUNCTIONING. See pages 45 to 47.)

ACTIVITY PLAN 2: UNDERSTANDING

PURPOSE OF ACTIVITY: To provide basic information about arthritis, diabetes, and Parkinson's disease and the importance of exercise in treating these conditions.

DESCRIPTION OF ACTIVITY: The leader and the elder will read together information about arthritis, diabetes, and Parkinson's disease, look over the exercises to note whether any are not recommended for the elder, and prepare for the next session.

BENEFITS OF ACTIVITY: As well as providing basic information about these conditions, the tips and information may encourage confidence to exercise daily.

BEFORE THE SESSION:

Things to do

The leader will read through the activity plan and Appendix C to become familiar with information provided. Following the guidelines of the program training manual, the elder's doctor should be provided a copy of the exercise illustrations from Appendix C and asked to indicate which exercises, if any, are not safe for the elder.

Things to take

Exercise illustrations from Appendix C

WHAT TO DO DURING THE SESSION:

Greeting and opening chat; pay attention to any immediate needs.

Complete any unfinished business from previous session.

Explain the session's activities.

Do activities.

The elder and leader may read and discuss the following:

The more we have learned about the human body, the more we have come to recognize the importance of physical activity. For many people the word "exercise" is not a pleasant one, but the fact remains that some form of exercise is needed on a daily basis to keep the body mobile. This is true for everyone--young or old, healthy or not. Exercise combined with a healthy diet and life-style can prevent many illnesses. It is also prescribed after an illness to help bring the body back to normal and, in some cases, during ongoing illnesses to prevent a condition from becoming worse.

Arthritis, diabetes, and Parkinson's disease affect many older people. In all three cases, being inactive and overweight worsens the condition, and in all three cases, exercise is a very important part of treatment.

1. OSTEOARTHRITIS

There are two major types of arthritis: osteoarthritis and rheumatoid arthritis. It is important to know the difference because they need different medical management. Both respond to proper exercise at the proper time.

Osteoarthritis is the most common form of arthritis. Most elderly people are affected to some degree by this condition. Basically, it is the wearing out of the joint, which has been under abnormal strain. Some occupations require the use of one or more joints continually. This type of repetitive action can bring about arthritis.

In the majority of cases, arthritis is in the weight-bearing joints (back, hips, and knees), which are subjected to a great deal of work over a lifetime. Being overweight puts even more strain on the joints.

The main symptoms are pain, muscle weakness, and deformity. The condition cannot be cured, but relief is possible. Treatment includes the following:

a. Weight reduction (to reduce pain and swelling)
b. Simple exercises (to strengthen muscles, prevent stiffness, and discourage deformity)
c. Basic anti-inflammatory drugs (to reduce pain and swelling)

d. Application of heat (to reduce pain and relax the muscles, enabling fuller movement)

In using heat, care should be taken to avoid burning the skin; a warm temperature is better than very hot because discomfort could cause the muscle to spasm, thereby undoing the benefit of relaxing. Gentle massage or rubbing produces warmth and is included in these exercises to help warm up muscles prior to moving them.

2. RHEUMATOID ARTHRITIS

Rheumatoid arthritis is a chronic disease involving many joints over a number of years. No age group is exempt although it most commonly appears in the thirties to fifties. Women are affected three times as often as men. The onset is usually gradual, beginning in the small joints of the hands and feet and moving to the larger ones; hips usually are not involved.

The pain that comes with rheumatoid arthritis is almost constant but is very acute during "flare-ups." In the acute stage, hospitalization is sometimes necessary; rest, good diet, and doctor's treatment are important. After the flare-up subsides, a therapist can begin to move the joints gently. At this stage do not exercise unless with the guidance of a physical therapist, as it is easy to damage the joints further. Once the person is stronger and back home, daily exercises are recommended to prevent weakness and deformity.

Tips for exercising with arthritis:

a. Do the exercises slowly and carefully. It is important that each movement is taken as far as the joint will go and a <u>tiny</u> bit farther. The number of times an exercise is done is less important than the full range of motion achieved. With osteoarthritis a certain amount of pain can be tolerated while exercising; joints affected by rheumatoid arthritis, however, should <u>not</u> be moved when inflamed.
b. Strengthen the muscles. As muscles gradually strengthen, increase the number of repetitions. This is important because muscles hold the joints in the proper position. For muscles that have become <u>very</u> weak, simply moving the limbs and contracting the muscles (tightening them) will gradually strengthen them. As strength increases, move on to the unit called "strength exercises," which adds a litle more resistance to make the muscle work harder and thereby become stronger.
c. Exercise daily. It is a fact that muscles and bones lose strength when inactive. This is true of healthy athletes, physically limited individuals, or anyone of normal health. The body must be used in order to keep it functioning properly.

3. DIABETES

There are two basic types of diabetes: insulin-dependent and non-insulin-dependent. Insulin-dependent diabetics are usually under 20 years of age at the onset of the disease, and the symptoms appear suddenly and progress rapidly. They constitute less than 10 percent of the diabetic population. Non-insulin-dependent (or adult-onset) diabetics are usually over 40 years of age at the onset of the disease, have a history of diabetes in the family, and make up 90 percent of the diabetic population. Symptoms appear and develop slowly.

Although not curable today, diabetes is largely controllable. Optimal treatment involves balancing three things: diet, insulin, and exercise. The well-regulated adult-onset diabetic can anticipate a near normal life expectancy and life-style. For the juvenile-onset or insulin-dependent diabetic, treatment is more complicated but still manageable. The presence of the disease over many years affects the blood vessels, which in turn affect the vision, kidneys, and heart, making proper diagnosis very important.

Exercise plays an important role in both types of diabetes. In order to know just which kind of exercise program to begin with, it is important to know whether or not the diabetic has vascular complications. Dr. Robert Cantu, in his book Diabetes and Exercise, states that diabetics without vascular complications may undertake a regular adult fitness program, and those with vascular complications should begin with a cardiac rehabilitation exercise program to build up their strength fully under the guidance of a physician. Both will benefit greatly from exercise.

Diabetics usually work very closely with their physicians to control their condition. The diabetic who exercises must plan when to exercise, when to administer insulin, and what to do in case of low blood sugar. Although the exercises in this unit are designed to be safe for anyone, the diabetic is asked to consult with a physician about doing them and make it clear that the exercises focus on flexibility and relaxation to promote better circulation and help strengthen very weak muscles.

Tips for exercising diabetics

a. Have an emergency supply of sugar handy. Life-savers or other hard candy made with corn syrup enter the blood stream faster than chocolate.
b. Be aware of the times of day an insulin reaction is likely to occur and how long you can go without refueling your sugar supply.
c. If the signal of low blood sugar comes while exercising, stop immediately and drink sugary beverages or take honey or candy.
d. Extreme hot or cold weather and infections cause the body to work harder and expend more energy (burn more sugar). This requires an adjustment of insulin or caloric intake beforehand.

e. For the insulin-dependent, the injection site should be in a part of the body that will not be exercised.
f. Exercise with someone else present.

4. PARKINSON'S DISEASE

Parkinson's disease is caused by a malfunction in a special part of the brain that controls voluntary movement (such as walking, chewing, smiling, etc.). It comes on so gradually that friends and relatives are not aware of the changes taking place. It is more common in men than women and usually comes on between the ages of 50 and 65.

Muscles become rigid and movement is slow and stiff. Rigidity of the muscles interferes with circulation resulting in pain and fatigue. Even throat and facial muscles can be affected. Until the very advanced stages of the disease, the mind is not affected, so the person sees, feels, and experiences all that is going on.

All treatment is directed toward relief of discomfort and prolonging activity. Physical therapy treatments done a few times a week at the hospital are not enough. In order to maintain what is gained there, the person with Parkinson's disease should work at home or in a support group to improve or to prevent further stiffening and limitation of movement.

The major muscles that have tightened (shortened) are those that cause the back, hips, knees, arms, and hands to bend. This creates a stooped posture; walking becomes a shuffle, and stopping and starting become difficult. Exercises should focus on improving circulation, relaxing, stretching and strengthening the muscles, and keeping range of motion in the joint.

Many people always feel cold due to lack of movement and poor circulation, which causes even more stiffness. The person with Parkinson's disease would benefit greatly from learning to relax and breathe deeply, and working toward straightening the bent limbs (the back, hips, knees, arms, and hands). Exercises in this unit as well as those in other units, would be useful.

<u>Tips for exercising with Parkinson's disease</u>

a. The number of times an exercise is done is not as important as the full range of movement.
b. Exercise twice a day. Some exercises can be done at odd times throughout the day, especially those for the feet and hands, shoulders, neck.
c. Focus on correcting the posture by stretching and bending, which counteracts the bent or stooped posture. Straighten the back, legs, and arms.
d. Work slowly and try to breathe fully to improve circulation.
e. Work on skid-proof surfaces, using a chair for support.

Session wrap-up; enjoy a snack if desired.

During this time review the exercise illustrations from Appendix C. The leader can demonstrate a few exercises that will be used in future sessions.

ENDING THE SESSION:

Share the basket.

Talk about and confirm next session.

AFTER THE SESSION:

Write up comments.

IDEAS FOR MODIFYING THE ACTIVITY:

TIPS FOR SAFETY:

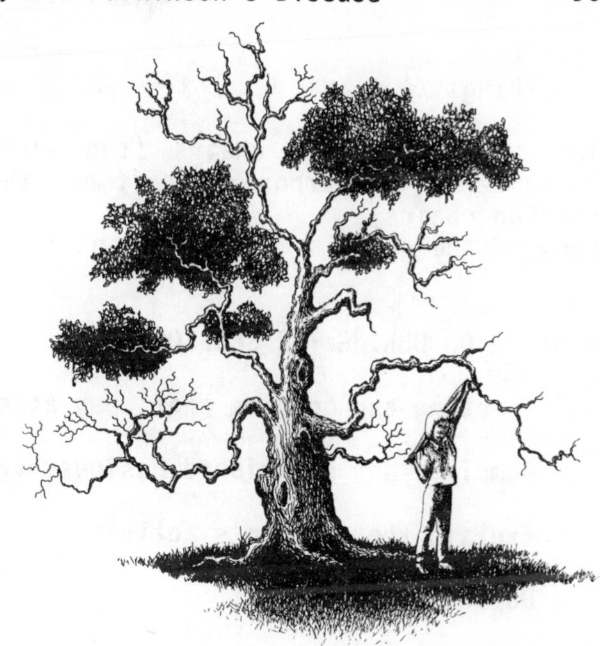

UNIT NAME: Exercises for Arthritis, Diabetes and Parkinson's Disease

ACTIVITY PLAN 3: MASSAGING AND STRETCHING

PURPOSE OF ACTIVITY: To experience the calming and revitalizing effects of stretching and relaxing by learning to stretch and breathe effectively. To develop an awareness of one's body and the ability to control it. To increase circulation and flexibility in joints throughout the body.

DESCRIPTION OF ACTIVITY: The leader will guide the elder through a light and simple self-massage, introduce the basics of gently stretching and shaking out muscles to release tension, and encourage the elder to feel comfortable about moving.

BENEFITS OF ACTIVITY: This session will allow the elder and leader to become acquainted while doing some simple activities that will help the leader to evaluate further the needs and special interests of the elder. Interaction is important to overcoming initial timidity about exercising.

BEFORE THE SESSION:

Things to do

Read the activity plan and the unit exercise illustrations in Appendix C to become familiar with the exercises. Make sure the doctor's approval of the exercise unit has been completed.

Things to take

Two sturdy, armless chairs (the elder may have kitchen chairs that would serve the purpose, but if not the leader may have to bring sturdy folding chairs)
Copy of the exercise illustrations from Appendix C

WHAT TO DO DURING THE SESSION:

Greeting and opening chat; pay attention to any immediate needs.

Complete any unfinished business from previous session.

Explain the session's activities.

Do activities.

Use the exercises provided for this unit (Appendix C). Do these exercises. Numbers refer to the location of the exercises in the appendix.

2. Massage
32. Whole body stretches
4. Rag doll

Session wrap-up; enjoy a snack if desired.

ENDING THE SESSION:

Share the basket.

Talk about and confirm next session.

Emphasize the importance of moving body parts to prevent stiffness and improve circulation. Encourage the elder to do some stretching and massaging during the coming week to prevent soreness and stiffness. Stress the importance of doing gentle activity throughout the day. Explain that the next session will include flexibility exercises for the neck, torso, legs, and feet.

AFTER THE SESSION:

Write up comments.

IDEAS FOR MODIFYING THE ACTIVITY:

TIPS FOR SAFETY: Activities during this session are purposely light and simple. This will enable the leader and the elder to evaluate their needs and make any necessary adjustments for future sessions. Important points to remember:

1. Move slowly. For some frail elderly, moving rapidly can produce cardiovascular stress. Heavy breathing and flushing are signs that the individual is working beyond safe limits. Stop activity and allow the individual to rest. You may want to stop exercising for that session and try working at a slower pace next time. It is important that the individual learn what is safe to do so as not to assume that <u>all</u> activity is ruled out.

2. Breathe regularly throughout these activities. Holding the breath increases blood pressure and puts a strain on the heart.

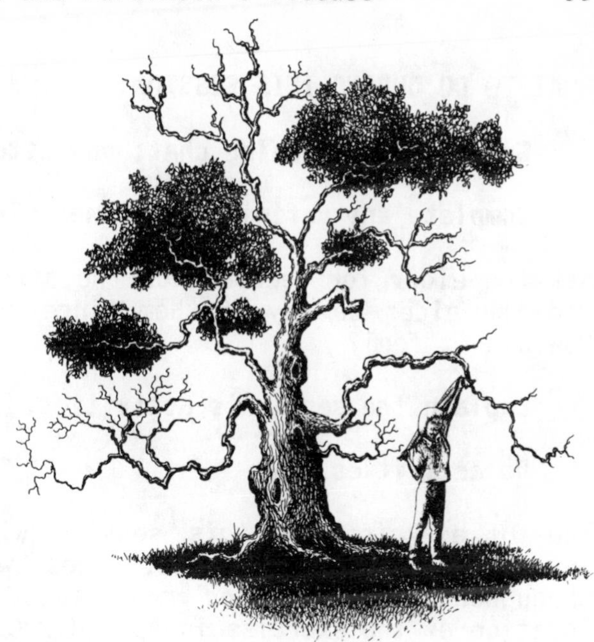

UNIT NAME: Exercises for Arthritis, Diabetes, and Parkinson's Disease

ACTIVITY PLAN 4: MOVING THE MAJOR BODY PARTS

PURPOSE OF ACTIVITY: To reinforce body awareness and add new exercises for the neck, shoulders, torso, legs, and feet.

DESCRIPTION OF ACTIVITY: The leader will lead the elder through the massage and relaxation activities and then demonstrate and lead flexibility exercises using the major body parts.

BENEFITS OF ACTIVITY: Each session will build on the previous one so that there will be a series of familiar exercises each week. Repetition will help to build confidence, as well as serve as a reference point for improvement over time.

WHAT THE ELDER WILL DO: The elder will follow the leader through last week's stretch and relaxation exercises and perform 2 repetitions each of the 7 new exercises.

BEFORE THE SESSION:

Things to do

Read the activity plan and try out the exercises.

Things to take

Exercise illustrations from Appendix C

WHAT TO DO DURING THIS SESSION:

Greeting and opening chat; pay attention to any immediate needs.

Complete any unfinished business from previous session.

Ask the elder for feedback on the stretching and relaxation activities. Did the elder do any of them since the last session? What was tried? How did it feel?

Explain the session's activities.

Do activities.

The 10 exercises in this session will include basic movements that involve the major body parts. These will help to stimulate circulation throughout the body and move major joints. Numbers refer to the location of the exercise in Appendix C.

2. Massage
4. Rag doll
5. Neck
6. Shoulder shrugs
15. Torso twist
17. Legs
18. Walk-in-place
19. Ankle rotation
32. Whole body stretches
33. Shake out

Session wrap-up; enjoy a snack if desired.

Discuss with the elder which of the exercises felt best. Which would he/she like to do during the week? Discuss what times of the day some of these activities could be done easily. Point out that some of these can be done on the edge of the bed or while watching television, listening to the radio, or talking on the phone. Relate the movements done in these exercises to daily activities.

ENDING THE SESSION:

Share the basket.

Talk about and confirm next session.

AFTER THE SESSION:

Write up comments.

IDEAS FOR MODIFYING THE ACTIVITY: All of the exercises in this session are done seated. Once they become familiar, depending on the strength of the individual, the elder and leader can vary the routine by doing some seated and some standing.

TIPS FOR SAFETY: Safety precautions are the same for each session. Move slowly and carefully. Monitor for signs of cardiovascular stress: heavy breathing and flushing. INDIVIDUALS WHO HAVE HAD A HIP REPLACED SHOULD AVOID BRINGING THE KNEE UP ANY CLOSER TO THE CHEST THAN 90°, WHICH IS THE ANGLE MADE BETWEEN THE TORSO AND THE THIGHS WHEN IN A NORMAL SEATED POSITION.

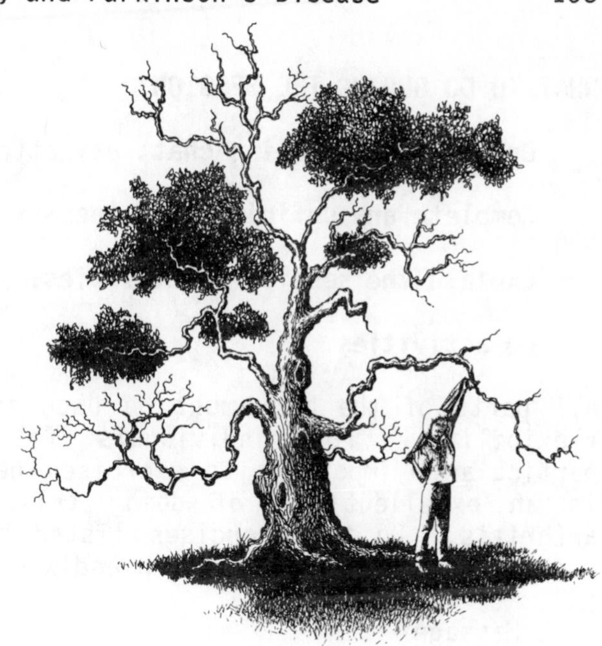

UNIT NAME: Exercises for Arthritis, Diabetes, and Parkinson's Disease

ACTIVITY PLAN 5: THE GOOD MORNING STRETCH

PURPOSE OF ACTIVITY: To go over exercises from the previous session and provide additional exercises that will involve larger body motions.

DESCRIPTION OF ACTIVITY: The leader will follow the previous sequence of exercises to help establish a routine. Five new exercises will be included in the appropriate places: the "good morning" stretch, side stretches, shoulder rolls, leg lifts, and facial exercises. The elder will perform 2 or 3 repetitions of exercises with the leader.

BENEFITS OF ACTIVITY: The leader will help to establish rhythms for the various exercises that are appropriate for the elder. Rhythms are kept very slow to enable full movements and also to avoid heart strain. All exercises may be done seated.

BEFORE THE SESSION:

Things to do

Read the activity plan to become familiar with the exercises.

Things to take

Exercise illustrations from Appendix C

WHAT TO DO DURING THE SESSION:

Greeting and opening chat; pay attention to any immediate needs.

Complete any unfinished business from previous session.

Explain the session's activities.

Do activities.

All parts of the body must be used in order to maintain strength and flexibility. For individuals with Parkinson's disease it is particularly important to exercise the facial muscles. "Making faces" is an excellent way of doing this. Jaws are also susceptible to arthritis. Do the exercises listed below. The number refers to the location of the exercise in Appendix C.

2. Massage
3. Face
4. Rag doll
5. Neck
6. Shoulder shrugs
7. Shoulder rolls
8. Good morning stretch
15. Torso twist
16. Side stretches
17. Legs
18. Walk-in-place
19. Ankle rotations
32. Whole body stretches
33. Shake out

Session wrap-up; enjoy a snack if desired.

Discuss today's activities. If any of the activities need to be modified, discuss ways of doing this. Introduce the new activity for next session: "Next week we are going to give special attention to feet." Ask the elder to think about something to share that pertains to feet. This can be in the form of facts, humorous anecdotes, songs, poems, or graphics.

ENDING THE SESSION:

Share the basket.

Talk about and confirm next session.

AFTER THE SESSION:

Write up comments.

IDEAS FOR MODIFYING THE ACTIVITY:

TIPS FOR SAFETY: Move slowly and carefully. Monitor for signs of cardiovascular stress: flushing and heavy breathing. Stop if the elder shows any of these signs or is experiencing pain anywhere.

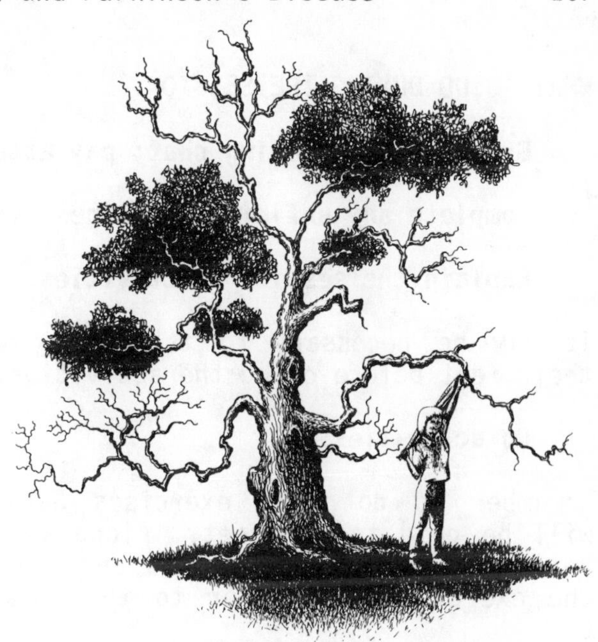

UNIT NAME: Exercises for Arthritis, Diabetes, and Parkinson's Disease

ACTIVITY PLAN 6: ATTENDING TO FEET

PURPOSE OF ACTIVITY: To focus attention on feet and perform exercises that will promote strength, balance, and coordination and improve circulation in the legs and feet.

DESCRIPTION OF ACTIVITY: The leader will lead the elder through 2 or 3 repetitions of the exercises and share information about feet with the elder.

BENEFITS OF ACTIVITY: This session will give the elder an opportunity to share with the leader, in a slightly different way, something that can be serious or whimsical or both. This is an exercise in positive thinking, to direct focus away from aches and pains. All exercises in this session may be done seated.

BEFORE THE SESSION:

Things to do

Read the activity plan and look for information on feet.

Things to take

A cylinder suitable for using as a foot massager, such as a rolling pin or plastic bottle that can be placed on the floor.

Anecdotes, facts, songs, poems, and the like about feet.

Illustrations from Appendix C.

WHAT TO DO DURING THE SESSION:

Greeting and opening chat; pay attention to any immediate needs.

Complete any unfinished business from previous session.

Explain the session's activities.

It may be necessary to take time for the leader and elder to wash their feet before doing the activities.

Do activities.

Remember to do these exercises S-L-O-W-L-Y. Some special attention will be paid to the feet. Along with the other exercises, these will help to improve circulation and mobility. The numbers in front of the exercise names refer to the location of the exercise in Appendix C.

1. Special: Salute to "Feet!" A time to share information about feet and do some additional activities. If at all possible, remove your shoes to do the following:

    21. Toe wiggles
    23. Inchworm
    22. Foot curls
    20. Heel and toe lifts
    24. The Charleston

2. If possible, hand-rub your feet:

    a. Hold all of the toes of one foot in one hand and move them all up and down.
    b. Rub the ball of the foot and the arches, using the knuckles of your hands.
    c. Rub gently around the ankle bones with your finger tips.
    d. Knead the heel of your foot.
    e. Gently pull and twist each toe.
    f. Gently slap the balls and soles of your feet.
    g. Place cylinder on the floor. Roll it back and forth with your feet gently massaging the soles and heels.

3. Put shoes and/or socks back on, walk around and see how those new feet feel! Remember to prop them up once in a while and give them a rest.

4. Discuss some pointers about footwear:

    a. While exercising, wear flexible shoes to get the most range of motion.
    b. Shoes protect and support the feet but often are so tight that they restrict motion as well as circulation.

c. Stockings too are sometimes so tight that they cramp the toes and restrict motion.
d. Toes are important for balancing. Walking is important for circulation, and good circulation is important to your health.

Session wrap-up; enjoy a snack if desired.

Discuss today's exercises. Talk about next week's special activity and how to prepare for that session. The focus next week will be on shoulders and hands.

ENDING THE SESSION:

Share the basket.

Talk about and confirm next session.

The next session will be on hands, arms, and shoulders. Encourage the elder to bring an anecdote about hands.

AFTER THE SESSION:

Write up comments.

IDEAS FOR MODIFYING THE ACTIVITY:

TIPS FOR SAFETY: As with all sessions in this unit, move slowly and carefully. Monitor for signs of overdoing: heavy breathing, flushing, and dizziness are all signs to stop and rest.

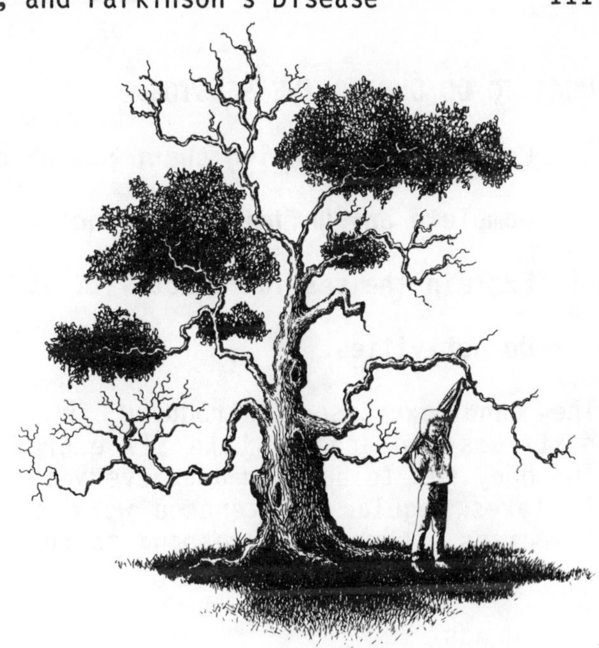

UNIT NAME: Exercises for Arthritis, Diabetes and Parkinson's Disease

ACTIVITY PLAN 7: SHOULDERS, ARMS, AND HANDS

PURPOSE OF ACTIVITY: To perform exercises and pay special attention to shoulders, arms, and hands. To continue to encourage positive thoughts and focus on positive happenings.

DESCRIPTION OF ACTIVITY: The leader will begin the activities with the hands and proceed through the routine, adding new flexibility exercises for the shoulders and arms. The session will close with sharing information about hands, arms, and shoulders. Do 2 to 3 repetitions of each exercise.

BENEFITS OF ACTIVITY: This session allows the elder to contribute information that has something to do with the activities of the hands, arms, shoulders.

BEFORE THE SESSION:

Things to do

Read the activity plan and try out the new exercises.

Things to take

Small bean bags or sponges, 1 or 2 per person
Scarf or light towel for each person
Additional information about hands, arms, and shoulders
Illustrations from Appendix C

WHAT TO DO DURING THE SESSION:

Greeting and opening chat; pay attention to any immediate needs.

Complete any unfinished business from previous session.

Explain the session's activities.

Do activities.

The hand exercises introduced in this session will help to reduce stiffness and aches. Like all exercises, they must be done regularly. The body has to be warmed up everyday; like any good piece of machinery, it takes regular maintenance work to keep it going! Do the following exercises. Numbers correspond to the order of the exercises in Appendix C.

1. Hands
2. Massage
3. Face
4. Rag doll
5. Neck
6. Shoulder shrugs
7. Shoulder rolls
8. Good morning stretch
9. Palms up, palms down
10. Elbow bends
11. Elbow touches
12. Elbow circles
13. Arm circles
14. Scarf/towel
15. Torso twist
16. Side stretches
17. Legs
18. Walk-in-place
19. Ankle rotation
20. Heel and toe lifts
21. Toe wiggles
22. Foot curls
23. Inchworm
24. The Charleston

Session wrap-up; enjoy a snack if desired.

Share anecdotes about hands, shoulders, arms.

ENDING THE SESSION:

Share the basket.

Talk about and confirm next session.

The next session will include exercises and information for backs.

AFTER THE SESSION:

Write up comments.

IDEAS FOR MODIFYING THE ACTIVITY: The bean bags and scarves can be used in many creative ways. Explore the possibilities but take care to control the energy level to match the capabilities of the individual involved.

TIPS FOR SAFETY: Move slowly and carefully. Monitor for signs of overdoing. Make sure that bean bags, scarves, and towels do not get in the way of movements or force movement beyond the individual comfort zone.

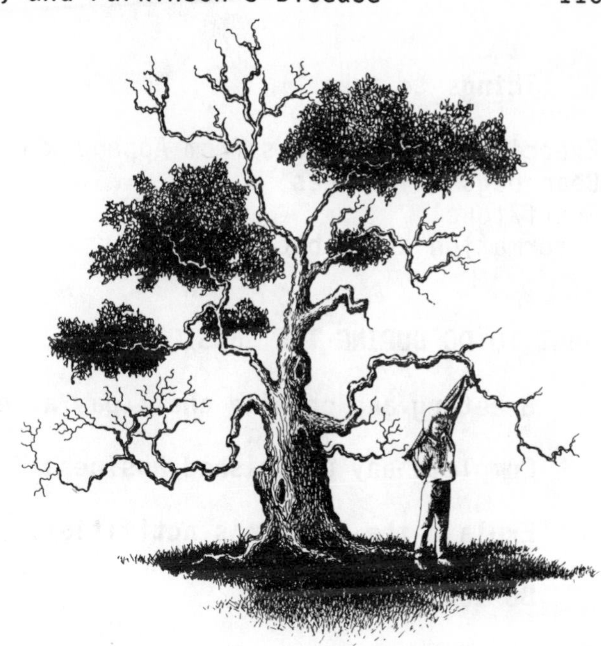

UNIT NAME: Exercises for Arthritis, Diabetes, and Parkinson's Disease

ACTIVITY PLAN 8: BACK EXERCISES

PURPOSE OF ACTIVITY: To continue with basic exercises while introducing new ones to promote flexibility and mobility. Special exercises will focus on the back.

DESCRIPTION OF ACTIVITY: The leader will lead the elder through the series of exercises from previous sessions and discuss special exercises that can be done for the back.

BENEFITS OF ACTIVITY: This session allows for sharing of information about the back.

WHAT THE ELDER WILL DO: The elder will perform 2 or 3 repetitions of the exercises from the series. Also, there will be some sharing of information about backs.

BEFORE THE SESSION:

Things to do

Read the activity plan to become familiar with new exercises. Gather information about back care. Call or visit a hospital, clinic, or doctor's office to pick up pamphlets on back care.

Things to take

Exercise illustrations from Appendix C
Bean bags or sponges
Scarf/towel
Information about backs

WHAT TO DO DURING THE SESSION:

Greeting and opening chat; pay attention to any immediate needs.

Complete any unfinished business from previous session.

Explain the session's activities.

Do activities.

Do the following exercises from previous sessions. Numbers associated with exercise names indicate location in Appendix C. The new activities in this session are to help release tight muscles and keep the spine flexible.

1. Hands
4. Rag doll
5. Neck
8. Good morning stretch
12. Elbow circles
14. Scarf/towel
15. Torso twist
16. Side stretches
18. Walk-in-place
21. Toe wiggles
23. Inchworm
24. The Charleston

1. Discuss the following ideas:

   a. Are there things that make your back "talk back"? What are they? How can they be prevented?
   b. Discuss principles of good posture for sitting and standing.
   c. Point out ways of lifting and moving objects that will protect the back.
   d. Point out ways of bending and reaching that will protect the back.

2. Do this special exercise designed to keep your back flexible:

   a. Sit erect, arms relaxed by your sides.
   b. Drop your head forward slightly, and slowly lower your head toward your knees.

c. Go down only as far as you comfortably can. Let your arms relax.
d. Slowly, straighten up your lower back, then your middle back, then your upper back, and last of all, straighten up your neck as you lift your chin from your chest.
e. Finish by lifting your face and chest up toward the ceiling and then bring your gaze back to some point straight ahead.
f. Caution: come up very S-L-O-W-L-Y to prevent dizziness.

3. Do these special exercises designed to be done from the floor or a firm bed or couch.

   a. Lie on your back with your knees bent, feet pulled up close to your buttocks. Rest your arms across your chest or on your stomach and breathe and relax in this position for a few minutes (five minutes is adequate and more won't hurt a bit!). This simple exercise releases tension in the lower back by allowing the muscles to lengthen from their contracted position of standing. Just imagine those tight muscles melting like butter on the firm floor or mattress!
   b. Lie on your back and bring one knee up to your chest, holding it there with your hands, then bring the other leg up and hold it up to your chest. This one also helps those lower back muscles (NOT RECOMMENDED FOR PERSONS WHO HAVE UNDERGONE HIP REPLACEMENT).
   c. On your hands and knees, arch your back up like a cat stretching; let your back drop down in a reverse arch, swayback fashion. Now look back over one shoulder and then the other.
   d. To get out of bed with the least amount of strain on your back, avoid sitting straight up from the prone position. Instead, roll over onto your side close to the edge of the bed, use your arms to brace yourself and push yourself up, swing your legs gently over the edge of the bed and onto the floor. Sit there on the edge of the bed for a few moments. You may also want to use this time to do some breathing exercises or neck and feet exercises to get your motor going before you stand up.

Session wrap-up; enjoy a snack if desired.

ENDING THE SESSION:

Share the basket.

Talk about and confirm next session.

AFTER THE SESSION:

Write up comments.

IDEAS FOR MODIFYING THE ACTIVITY: Some days are more energetic than others. Always feel free to cut the amount of time or leave out particular exercises if there is pain in a specific part of the body, but try to do what can be done. Remember the "use it or lose it" admonition!

TIPS FOR SAFETY: Monitor for the signs of cardiovascular stress throughout the session. Always modify the pace or energy level to be within safe bounds. If the elder does not care to get down on the floor for the back exercises, or if the elder has not tried getting up from the floor in a long time, then do not encourage floor work. It is safer to use a firm couch or bed for these exercises.

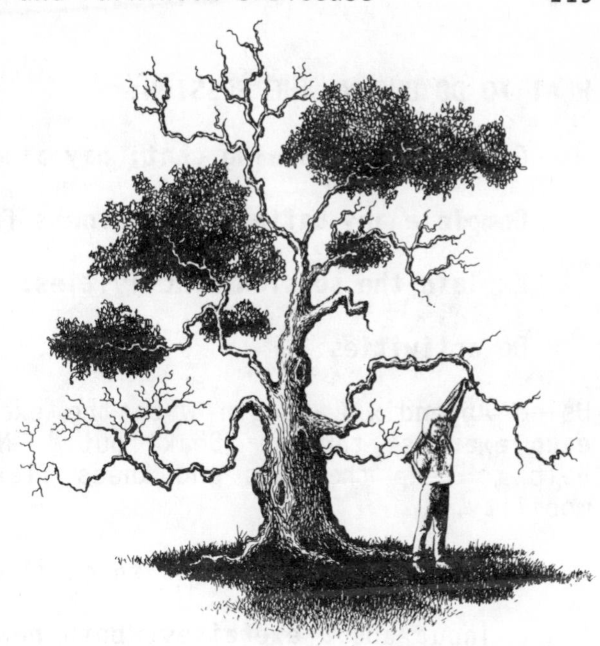

UNIT NAME: Exercises for Arthritis, Diabetes, and Parkinson's Disease

ACTIVITY PLAN 9: MORE LEG EXERCISES

PURPOSE OF ACTIVITY: To continue to do the basic exercises with additional exercises for the hips, legs, and knees.

DESCRIPTION OF ACTIVITY: The leader will lead the elder through all the previous exercises. New exercises will be incorporated into the sequence to complete the exercises in Appendix C. Because of the number of exercises now involved in the session, repetitions are kept to two or three.

BENEFITS OF ACTIVITY: This session focuses on the lower body and thus will enable more standing activities if the elder is able to do them.

BEFORE THE SESSION:

Things to do

Read the activity plan and try out the new exercises.

Things to take

Exercise illustrations from Appendix C
Bean bags or sponges
Scarf/towel

WHAT TO DO DURING THE SESSION:

Greeting and opening chat; pay attention to any immediate needs.

Complete any unfinished business from previous session.

Explain the session's activities.

Do activities.

Using Appendix C, begin with the exercise "Hands" and continue doing each exercise through "Shake out." New exercises using the legs will help to keep the hips and knees flexible and improve circulation and mobility.

Session wrap-up; enjoy a snack if desired.

Share input about exercises, both new and old. The next session will have no new exercises.

ENDING THE SESSION:

Share the basket.

Talk about and confirm next session.

AFTER THE SESSION:

Write up comments.

IDEAS FOR MODIFYING THE ACTIVITY:

TIPS FOR SAFETY: Move slowly and carefully. Monitor for signs of stress: heavy breathing and flushing. When doing standing exercises, use chair back for support.

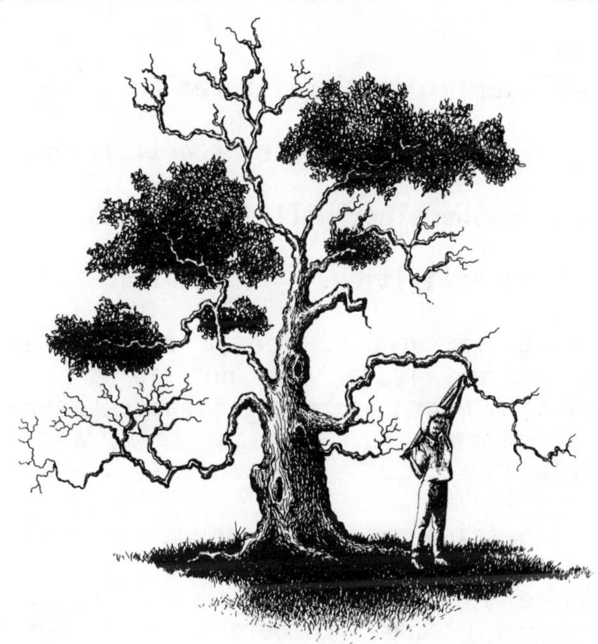

UNIT NAME: Exercises for Arthritis, Diabetes, and Parkinson's Disease

ACTIVITY PLAN 10: REVIEWING EXERCISES

PURPOSE OF ACTIVITY: To reinforce body memory and to help establish an exercise sequence that is easy to recall. To encourage the elder to lead the exercises.

DESCRIPTION OF ACTIVITY: There will be no new exercises added in this session; rather, attention will be focused on existing exercises, to become familiar with the feel and to make them flow together smoothly.

BENEFITS OF ACTIVITY: There is opportunity for personal expression and response in even the simplest exercises.

BEFORE THE SESSION:

Things to do

Things to take

Exercise illustrations from Appendix C
Bean bags or sponges
Scarf/towel

WHAT TO DO DURING THE SESSION:

Greeting and opening chat; pay attention to any immediate needs.

Complete any unfinished business from previous session.

Explain the session's activities.

Ask if the elder will be comfortable leading today's exercises.

Do activities.

Using Appendix C, repeat all the exercises in the appendix. If the elder and leader did not do all the exercises last session because of time, then begin the sequence where last session left off. Encourage the elder to use the appendix, and try to step out of the leadership role.

Session wrap-up; enjoy a snack if desired.

Share input about exercises. Leave Appendix C for the elder to use in the future. Encourage the elder to ask friends over and show them the exercises learned in this unit.

ENDING THE SESSION:

Share the basket.

Talk about and confirm next session.

AFTER THE SESSION:

Write up comments.

IDEAS FOR MODIFYING THE ACTIVITY:

TIPS FOR SAFETY: Move slowly and carefully. Monitor for signs of stress: heavy breathing and flushing. When doing standing exercises, use chair back for support.

REFERENCES AND RESOURCES

Cantu, R. Diabetes and exercise. New York: E. P. Dutton, 1982.

Caplow-Lindner, E., Harpay, L., & Samberg, S. Therapeutic dance movement. New York: Human Sciences Press, 1979.

Chrisman, D. Body recall. Berea, KY: Berea College Press, 1980.

Christensen, A., & Rankin, D. "Easy does it" yoga, for people over 60. Cleveland, OH: Saraswati Studio Press, 1975.

Corbin, D., & Metal-Corbin, J. Reach for it! Dubuque, IA: Eddie Bowers Publishing, 1983.

Hooker, S. Caring for elderly people. London: Routledge & Kegan Paul, 1976.

Lavigne, J. Home exercises for patients with Parkinson's disease. New York: The American Parkinson's Disease Association, 1978.

Letvin, M. Maggie's back book. Boston: Houghton Mifflin, 1976.

Rowe, J. W., & Besdine, R. W. Health and disease in old age. Boston: Little, Brown, 1982.

U.S. Department of Health, Education and Welfare. Working with older people: A guide to practice. Rockville, MD: U.S. Government Printing Office, 1978.

Wear, R. E. Fitness, vitality and you. Durham, NH: Council on Aging and New England Gerontology Center, University of New Hampshire, 1977.

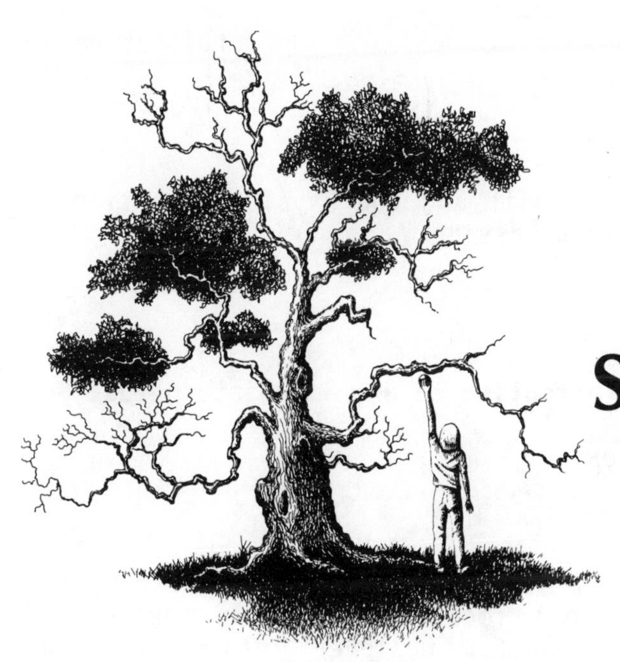

CHAPTER 8

Exercises for Special Purposes

UNIT NAME: Exercises for Special Purposes

(The first activity plan in all exercise units should be ASSESSING PHYSICAL FUNCTIONING. See pages 45 to 47.)

ACTIVITY PLAN 2: INTRODUCTION

PURPOSE OF ACTIVITY: To introduce general concepts of exercise which apply to the special purpose exercises in this unit.

DESCRIPTION OF ACTIVITY: The leader will go over the list of session names with the elder, then discuss which sessions are of special interest to the elder and why. The leader will then go over general concepts and precautions. The importance of flexibility, strength, balance, and agility for maintaining mobility and independence will be stressed.

BENEFITS OF ACTIVITY: This session will give the elder and leader an opportunity to become familiar with the session plans and decide which special exercises he/she may be interested in learning about and doing. The leader can use this time to identify special problems the elder may have in performing tasks of daily living. The tests of physical functioning completed in the first session will provide information about these needs. This will aid in selecting activities that are helpful in overcoming those difficulties.

BEFORE THE SESSION:

Things to do

The leader should read over the activity plans to become familiar with the material covered. Following the guidelines of the program, the elder's doctor should be provided a copy of the activity plans and asked to indicate which exercises, if any, are not safe for the elder.

Things to take

Copies of the activity plans in this unit and the Physical Functioning Assessment Record Sheet from the first session

WHAT TO DO DURING THE SESSION:

Greeting and opening chat; pay attention to any immediate needs.

Explain the session's activities.

Do activities.

1. The leader's introductory comments should point out that the exercises in each of the sessions focus on improving the use of particular body parts which are, for whatever reason, limited. Quite often, arthritis is the limiting factor, and it need not be. Gentle exercise is recommended for most kinds of arthritis. Other times it is simply inactivity that brings about stiffness and weakness in joints and muscles. These sessions cover the following:

   Shoulder and arm flexibility
   Exercises for hip replacements
   Care of the neck
   Flexibility and strength for feet and ankles
   Hand flexibility and strength
   Relaxation exercises
   Exercises for bladder control

2. These sessions do not have to be done in any particular order. All of the sessions need not be done. The elder and leader may decide to do only the session plans that pertain to special problems one or both experience. Session plans that target areas of need can be repeated in several sessions.

3. Although these exercises focus on particular problems, they are by no means limited to persons with problems. On the contrary, they are excellent for maintaining use of the body and are recommended for everyone as a means of preventing problems.

4. The following concepts are important:

   a. Being immobile, even for a short period of time, results in some slowing down of circulation and loss of strength, flexibility, range of motion, and balance, all of which are important in walking and carrying out the daily activities of life.
   b. One session includes exercises to be done when forced to stay in bed and stresses the importance of moving even when bedridden.

c. Move only within a comfortable range. Do not force any movement to the point of pain. STOP if experiencing pain and do not continue that particular movement until a physician is consulted. Do continue to do the movements that can be done without pain, to maintain strength and flexibility. Remember the phrase "Use it or lose it."

5. After looking at the activity plans in this unit, decide which activity plan to begin with next session.

Session wrap-up; enjoy a snack if desired.

ENDING THE SESSION:

Share the basket.

Talk about and confirm next session.

Make sure the doctor's approval of the activities in this unit is obtained before the next session.

AFTER THE SESSION:

IDEAS FOR MODIFYING THE ACTIVITY:

TIPS FOR SAFETY:

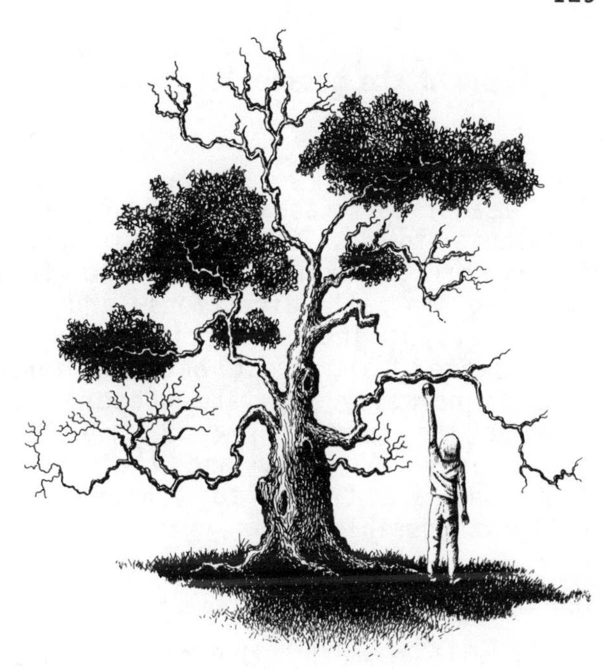

UNIT NAME: Exercises for Special Purposes

ACTIVITY PLAN 3: REACH FOR IT!

PURPOSE OF ACTIVITY: To provide basic exercises that will help improve and maintain the range of motion necessary to comb hair, put on and take off tops or coats and sweaters, and reach for objects.

DESCRIPTION OF ACTIVITY: The leader will discuss with the elder difficulties he/she may be experiencing with particular movements involved in daily activities requiring reaching up, out, or around. The leader will then perform with the elder the 7 exercises for flexibility of the shoulders and arms.

BENEFITS OF ACTIVITY: The exercises in this session are good for maintaining range of motion and should be done on a continuing basis, once the elder is able to do them on his/her own.

BEFORE THE SESSION:

Things to do

The leader should read through the activity plan and become familiar with the topic and try the exercises beforehand.

Things to take

WHAT TO DO DURING THE SESSION:

Greeting and opening chat; pay attention to any immediate needs.

Complete any unfinished business from previous session.

Explain the session's activities.

Do activities.

The leader discusses with the elder what, if any, movements are difficult to do, like putting on a jacket, combing hair, or tucking in a shirt. Explain that the following exercises will help with reaching in all directions and when done regularly will improve flexibility. These exercises can be done standing or sitting. If done seated, sit erect but not tense, with feet flat on the floor. Breathe normally and take deeper breaths with the big reaches. Never disrupt the normal flow of air--it creates stress and tension which limit body movement, and that is just the opposite of what these exercises are trying to achieve. Move slowly, deliberately, and as fully as possible.

Arm forward and up:

Begin with arms by the sides. Slowly lift one arm forward and up overhead, keeping elbow straight. Slowly return arm to starting position, keeping elbow straight. Repeat with other arm. Try it again on each side.

Arm sideward and up:

Begin with arms by the sides and palms toward body. With elbow straight, raise one arm slowly sideward and up overhead, turning palm as arm comes up. Only go as far as is comfortable. Slowly return arm to starting position, turning palm inward. Repeat with other arm. Do it again on each side.

Elbow up:

Place palm of right hand on or near the back of the neck. Remove it from there and place it down by the waist. Then, place it on or near the lower part of the back. Repeat process using left hand. Repeat on each side.

Arm to back and across the body:

With arm straight out to the side at shoulder level, elbow straight, push arm gently back. Bring arm forward and reach across the front of the body toward the other shoulder, elbow slightly bent. Repeat using other arm. Do it again for both sides.

Shrugs:

Begin with arms down by the sides. Raise one shoulder toward the ear. Lower shoulder toward hip. Repeat. Begin on other side. Repeat on each side.

√ Elbow:

Begin with arm extended to the front, palm up. Bend elbow until fingertips touch shoulder. Straighten elbow. Repeat. Begin on other arm. Repeat on both sides.

√ Doorknob:

Grasp an imaginary doorknob and twist it open and closed two or three times. Do the same with the other hand.

Session wrap-up; enjoy a snack if desired.

ENDING THE SESSION:

Share the basket.

Talk about and confirm next session.

AFTER THE SESSION:

Write up comments.

IDEAS FOR MODIFYING THE ACTIVITY:

TIPS FOR SAFETY: Use a sturdy chair. Always stop a particular exercise movement if it causes pain. These should not be painful to do. Work through the movements slowly.

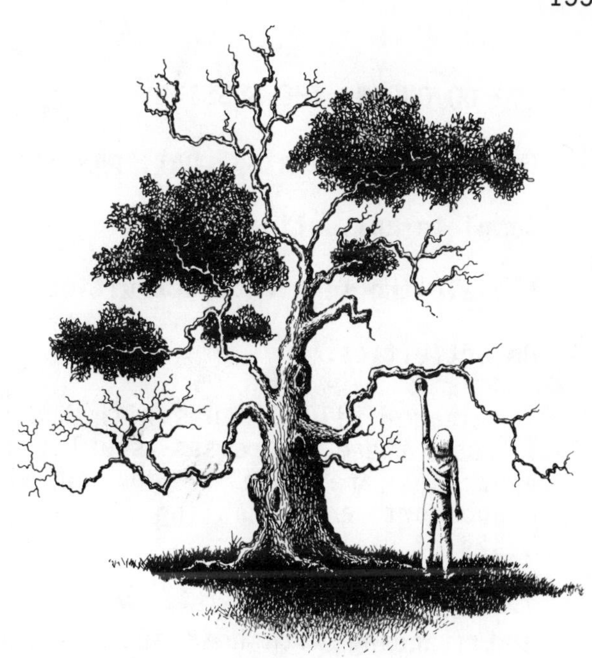

UNIT NAME: Exercises for Special Purposes

ACTIVITY PLAN 4: NECK CARE AND FLEXIBILITY

PURPOSE OF ACTIVITY: To discuss care of the neck and provide posture tips and flexibility exercises to enable pain-free daily activity. If the elder has osteoporosis, extreme movements should be avoided and these exercises are NOT recommended.

DESCRIPTION OF ACTIVITY: The leader will discuss the importance of good alignment (correct posture) and flexibility for preventing tension in the neck area. The elder and leader will go through flexibility exercises for the neck and the shoulders.

BENEFITS OF ACTIVITY: Almost everyone is prone to feel the effects of tension that accumulates in the neck and shoulders as a result of poor posture. Recognizing bad habits and correcting them throughout the day may help to eliminate the source of the problem and prevent soreness and stiffness while carrying on activities and hobbies.

BEFORE THE SESSION:

Things to do

The leader should read through the activity plan to become familiar with the topic to be discussed.

Things to take

WHAT TO DO DURING THE SESSION:

Greeting and opening chat; pay attention to any immediate needs.

Complete any unfinished business from previous session.

Explain the session's activities.

Do activities.

1. The leader will discuss with the elder if he/she has osteoporosis. If so, these exercises should not be done. If not, then these exercises are safe to do and will be very helpful in relieving discomfort and enabling freer movement while carrying out the tasks of daily living.

2. Try the following tips for correcting posture. Practice sitting and standing with head and shoulders straight but without tension. Sit with spine straight (no tension) and shoulders lined up over hips; not leaning forward or backward. Make sure shoulders are not pulled up toward ears or drooped forward. Check to see that the chin is not leading. Try jutting the chin out to see how it feels. Notice the front and back muscles of the neck tighten as the head is held that way. The chin should not be pulled in, military fashion. This creates a lot of unnecessary tension, too. Imagine being supported from above by a puppet string that lifts from the crown of the head. Feel the body grow in height. Maintaining this relaxed, balanced posture while seated or standing will help prevent fatigue.

3. The curve in the lower back (the lumbar curve) also has an effect on the upper back curve. If the lower back curves inward more than slightly, the upper back will curve outward to compensate--viewed from the side it is like a shallow "S" shape. Straightening up from the top of the head to the tip of the tailbone will help prevent neck and back pains. The back exercises included in the "Total hip exercises" session, which are done lying on the back, both strengthen and stretch the lower back muscles to lessen the lower back curve.

4. Do the following flexibility exercises while seated. These are very relaxing and may even cause drowsiness. Do them anytime. They are a pleasant break from daily tasks.

   a. Bring chin over toward right shoulder without lifting the shoulder. Bring chin over toward left shoulder. Repeat to left and right.

   b. Look straight ahead. Let head drop gently to the right side. Bring it back up to center. Let head drop gently to the left side. Bring it back up to center. Repeat to the left and right.

c. Push shoulders back, bring them up toward ears, and forward. Repeat this and then move them in the opposite direction by moving them forward, then up, then back and down. This will help to loosen the muscles that support the neck.

5. The following tips may help to protect the neck while sleeping:

While sleeping, the pillow should extend to just under the shoulders and should fill the space between the head and the bed just enough to maintain head position as if standing. In other words, no "crimp" in the neck. This also applies to lying on the back. Sleeping on the stomach is not good for the neck because it forces it into an extreme position, with the cheek against the bed.

Lying on the back with legs straight increases the curve in the lower back and is sometimes an uncomfortable position. Place a large pillow under the knees to lessen the curve and avoid strain on the lower back.

Use a firm mattress. A board placed under the mattress helps increase firmness and helps to reduce sag.

Choose the right pillow. Feather pillows are most adjustable and supportive. Polyester is the second best choice. Beware of pillows that may allow the head to drop backward, as both head and neck should be supported.

6. The following tips may help protect the neck while awake:

Avoid tilting the head back for long periods of time. Avoid tilting FAR back for even a short period of time. Bifocal eyeglasses force the wearer to tilt the head back under many close viewing conditions. Read below eye level but not too far below. Those who do much close work or reading should consider reading glasses or ask for a higher optical center in the reading segment of the bifocals. Avoid holding the head forward for long periods of time, such as when reading or writing.

7. Relaxation and neck health are affected by mental strain. The reduction of mental or emotional strain is one of the most important and effective ways to relieve neck strain and maintain overall health.

8. Practice the neck exercises regularly. A little self-discipline is required to avoid incorrect head and neck positions, but the effort will be worth it. The new habits will help reduce discomfort in the neck and shoulder region.

Session wrap-up; enjoy a snack if desired.

ENDING THE SESSION:

Share the basket.

Talk about and confirm next session.

AFTER THE SESSION:

Write up comments.

IDEAS FOR MODIFYING THE ACTIVITY:

TIPS FOR SAFETY: Exercises in this session plan should be done slowly and while seated. Discontinue if experiencing sharp pain. The elder's physician must approve this activity plan.

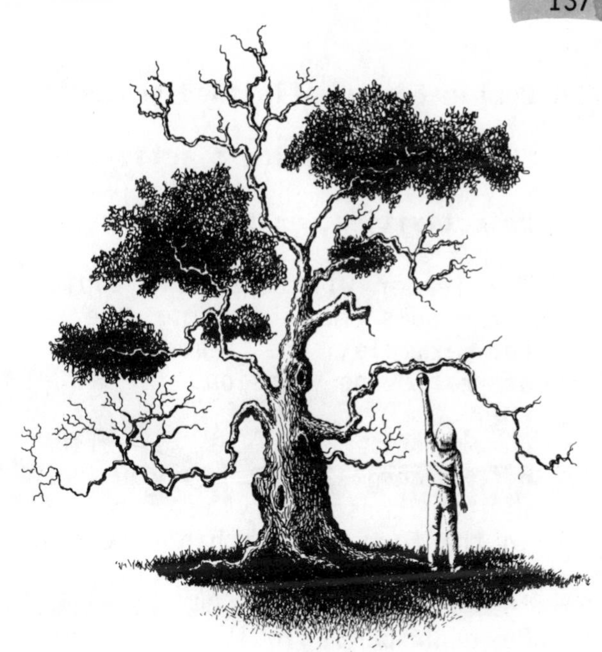

UNIT NAME: Exercises for Special Purposes

ACTIVITY PLAN 5: BREATHING AND RELAXATION

PURPOSE OF ACTIVITY: To practice breathing properly in order to relieve tension or stress and to promote relaxation.

DESCRIPTION OF ACTIVITY: The leader will discuss the role that stress or tension plays in making breathing difficult and inhibiting circulation and rest. The leader and elder will read through the instructions together. During the session they will practice breathing exercises and a muscle relaxation procedure.

BENEFITS OF ACTIVITY: The brief relaxation procedure described in this session is to be done seated, but it is helpful to practice in bed during sleepless nights. The breathing exercises strengthen the diaphragm and rib cage musculature.

BEFORE THE SESSION:

Things to do

The leader should read through the activity plan to become familiar with the topic.

Things to take

WHAT TO DO DURING THE SESSION:

Greeting and opening chat; pay attention to any immediate needs.

Complete any unfinished business from previous session.

Explain the session's activities.

Do activities.

1. The leader will open the topic with a discussion about individual techniques for handling the stress and strain of daily living. For example, the leader might say, "We each have our own ways of relieving tension. Have you found one or two things to do that work for you?" "Have you noticed yourself taking a deep breath after a stressful situation, be it good or bad? This is how the body naturally relieves tension, with a deep breath. We can consciously use this natural reaction to relieve tension in the form of breathing exercises."

2. The following are simple exercises to try. There are four parts. Do each part slowly so as not to become dizzy. (These exercises were adapted from Yoga Exercises for Every Body by Ruth Bender, Ruben Publishing, Avon, Connecticut, 1975.)

Part 1 - Abdominal Breathing:

Sit comfortably with a straight back. Now place your hands on your lower abdomen. Breathe in so that your hands move, not your upper chest. Breathe out and pull your stomach in. Repeat for two or three breaths. Make sure you breathe in quietly through your nose and out through your teeth with a hissing sound. Breathe slowly, as breathing fast often causes dizziness and faintness. Learn to control your breathing at all times. The out breath should be longer than the in breath. Once you develop a rhythm, set your own count. The out breath should take twice as long as the in breath. Gradually, over time, you will notice your breathing becoming deeper and fuller. The more relaxed you are, the deeper you breathe. Try this in bed sometime when sleep is difficult to find. Lie on your back with a pillow under your knees. This is the best position to promote relaxation. Just lie quietly and relax for a few moments, enjoying the still and quiet. Then practice a few deep breaths. This exercise works your diaphragm muscle.

Part 2 - Middle Ribcage Breathing:

Place your hands on your waist with thumbs pointing back and fingers forward. Slide your hands up your trunk until your fingers are on the sides of your chest, like ribs. Now inhale while feeling your hands move apart. Do not work the abdomen as in part 1, instead expand the ribcage. Release the air through your teeth as you press your hands together. Then take a few more breaths. This exercise strengthens the muscles of the ribcage.

Part 3 - Upper Ribcage Breathing:

Place your fingers on your collarbones and inhale as you raise your shoulders toward your ears. Feel the air rush in your nose without the help of your diaphragm or ribs. Relax and lower your shoulders, pressing down on your collarbones. Repeat for two more breaths.

Part 4 - The Total Breath:

Place your hands on your abdomen once more and begin inhaling, using only your diaphragm. Move your fingers to your ribcage and continue inhaling as your hands move apart. Finish the breath by moving your fingers to your collarbones and raising your shoulders. Now reverse the process and exhale S-L-O-W-L-Y while lowering your shoulders, then squeezing your hands together on your ribs, and finishing by pressing your hands against your abdomen. This accordion motion works all three ways we breathe. Repeat for three complete breaths.

3. Try this relaxation technique while lying on the floor, a couch, or a bed. To consciously relax each muscle group, lift one leg at a time a few inches off the bed and let it drop onto the bed completely relaxed. Lift arms up slightly off the bed and let them drop completely relaxed. Lift shoulders toward the ears in a shrug, and relax. Arch the back slightly, and relax. Lift the head from the pillow, and relax. Wrinkle the face hard, and relax.

Session wrap-up; enjoy a snack if desired.

ENDING THE SESSION:

Share the basket.

Talk about and confirm next session.

AFTER THE SESSION:

Write up comments.

IDEAS FOR MODIFYING THE ACTIVITY:

TIPS FOR SAFETY: Beginners sometimes hyperventilate and experience dizziness. Stop if this happens. Pace the breaths far apart and never progress when lightheadedness exists. While practicing during the session, sit in a firm chair with the feet flat on the floor, back straight, hands resting on the lower abdomen.

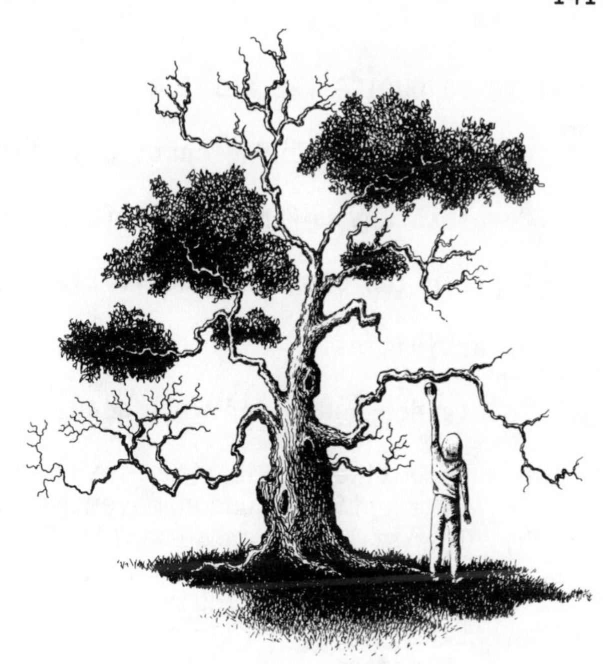

UNIT NAME: Exercises for Special Purposes

ACTIVITY PLAN 6: KEGEL EXERCISES FOR BLADDER CONTROL

PURPOSE OF ACTIVITY: To share useful advice concerning a common but often embarrassing disorder (incontinence). When the cause is explained, perhaps the individual will feel less self-conscious about the condition and will be more willing to try the exercises.

DESCRIPTION OF ACTIVITY: The leader will discuss with the elder the reasons for muscular weakness which lead to incontinence, and will outline the short list of Kegel exercises which tone and strengthen the muscles involved. The elder will follow instructions and attempt to feel the contractions of the muscles that surround the urethra and the anus.

BENEFITS OF ACTIVITY: As a result of childbirth and the natural aging process, some loss of tone in the muscles of the pelvic floor often occurs. This may cause incontinence. Many people afflicted with this annoying disorder may not be aware of the simple exercises which, when done correctly and consistently, can help to control urinary flow.

BEFORE THE SESSION:

Things to do

The leader should read through the activity plan to become familiar with the topic.

Things to take

WHAT TO DO DURING THE SESSION:

Greeting and opening chat; pay attention to any immediate needs.

Complete any unfinished business from previous session.

Explain the session's activities.

Do activities.

1. The leader and elder will read and discuss the following:

   a. Incontinence is the involuntary passage of urine brought on by exertion, sudden movement, coughing, sneezing, lifting.
   b. The strength and elasticity (ability to twitch, stretch, and contract) of the muscles that control the flow of urine are affected by childbirth, surgery, and the normal aging process.
   c. Like any other muscles, these respond to exercise. When the exercises are done correctly and consistently, the muscles involved gain tone and strength, and control of urination can be regained.

2. To gain an awareness of the muscles involved it is helpful to try to urinate small amounts at a time. One test to see if Kegel exercises are needed is to begin urination and consciously stop and start the flow three times. If this is impossible, the need to strengthen the muscles surrounding the urethra is evident. These Kegel exercises should be performed a minimum of three sessions a day (E. Noble, Essential Exercises for the Childbearing Years, Houghton Mifflin, Boston, 1976).

   a. To build tone, sit on a firm chair and contract the muscles as though stopping the flow of urine. Release. Start with 10 per session, increasing to 60 or more.
   b. Sit on a low stool or firm chair, knees apart, leaning forward slightly. Have someone there for support to get back up. Contract muscles in a wavelike tempo, starting in front and moving back toward and including the anus. Release in back and then in front. Start with 5 and increase as you are able. This exercise builds elasticity.
   c. Sit on the floor or bed with legs stretched out in front and back supported. Have someone there for support in getting down or up. Contract front to back as above. Hold strongly. Cross one ankle slowly over the other and uncross, maintaining pelvic floor tension. Then release back to front. Repeat with the other leg. Start with 6 repetitions and increase as you can. This exercise builds endurance.
   d. In any position, think of the pelvic floor as an elevator. Contract muscles a small amount at a time, as though rising to the next floor; continue to a level of 10. Release by coming down floor by floor, slowly. Tension is fully released when back to zero, not before or after. This exercise builds

conscious control. When possible, do 4 sets, and progress to the next exercise level.

e. Repeat the above exercise but force the elevator to return past the zero level. Apply pressure to force the pelvic floor to the basement or even lower. Gently contract back up to the street level and even up to the mezzanine. This is the level of habitual tension needed in the pelvic floor at all times.

Session wrap-up; enjoy a snack if desired.

ENDING THE SESSION:

Share the basket.

Talk about and confirm next session.

AFTER THE SESSION:

Write up comments.

IDEAS FOR MODIFYING THE ACTIVITY:

TIPS FOR SAFETY: It is important to point out that contracting a muscle in one part of the body does not require tensing the whole body or holding the breath. The person doing the exercises should pay attention to breathing normally. Holding the breath creates pressure and puts a strain on the heart. People with high blood pressure should be particularly careful to avoid the stress created by breath-holding.

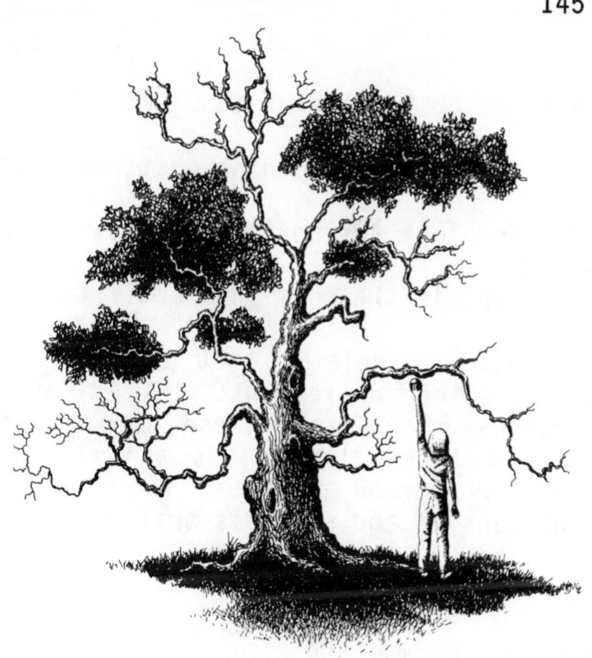

UNIT NAME: Exercises for Special Purposes

ACTIVITY PLAN 7: IN-BED FLEXIBILITY EXERCISES

PURPOSE OF ACTIVITY: To provide the elder with simple bed exercises to relieve back discomfort and muscle or joint stiffness which may develop from being in bed after a short bout with the flu or a cold.

DESCRIPTION OF ACTIVITY: The leader will introduce this session's topic and discuss the idea that even during short periods of illness, there is a need for relieving the discomfort of lying still. The leader and elder will read through the instructions and practice the exercises.

BENEFITS OF ACTIVITY: The exercises included in this session are useful for maintaining overall body strength and flexibility and a healthy back. They are particularly useful to an individual who must stay in bed for a period of time. Done gently, they can be performed while bedridden and continued afterward to regain and maintain strength and mobility. If getting up in the morning is difficult, these exercises can be done before getting out of bed.

BEFORE THE SESSION:

Things to do

The leader should read through the activity plan and try the exercises.

Things to take

WHAT TO DO DURING THE SESSION:

Greeting and opening chat; pay attention to any immediate needs.

Complete any unfinished business from previous session.

Explain the session's activities.

The leader explains that these exercises are worth doing and knowing about for two reasons: (1) to maintain strength, mobility, and a healthy lower back, these simple exercises should be done once a day and at least three times a week; and (2) if ill and confined to bed for any period of time, it is helpful to do some moving to relieve the tension and soreness that hours of lying still produce.

Do activities.

The elder may do these exercises while lying on the couch, floor, or bed. The leader may choose the floor to lie on while demonstrating.

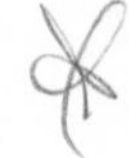

Pelvic Tilt:

Lie on your back with your knees bent and feet flat on the mat--you may wish to put a pillow under your knees, but it isn't necessary this time. Pull your stomach up and in. As you do this, let the small of your back flatten out against the floor or bed. Hold this position without tension. Keep breathing while doing this. This is excellent for relief of back discomfort and cannot be overdone; 5 to 10 minutes several times a day is recommended.

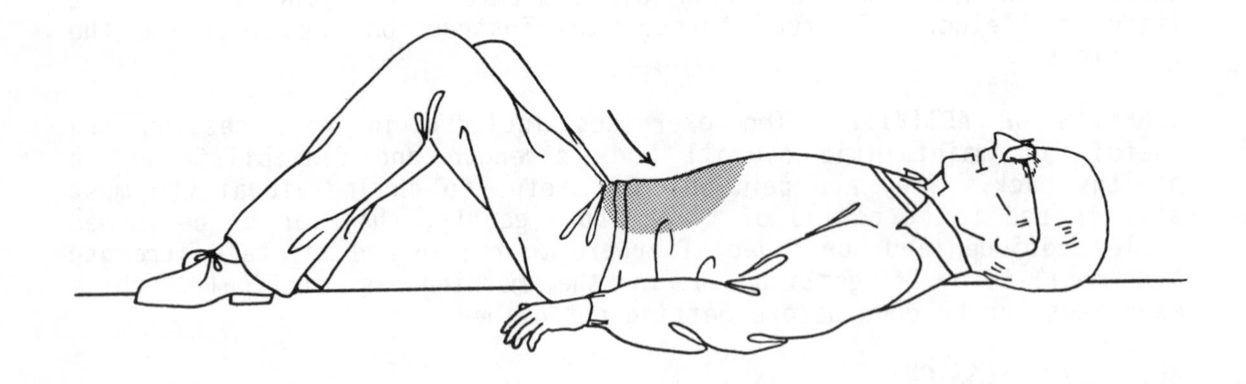

To do this seated, sit with your feet on the floor and back straight. Try to touch you waistband to the back of the chair.

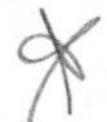

Knees to Chest (not recommended for persons with hip replacement):

Remain in the same position as in the previous exercise. Bring your left knee up to your chest. Hold it there with your hands. Don't force or pull; just hold it gently for 15 seconds while you practice steady, deep breathing. Repeat with the other leg. The next time you exercise, increase the amount of time you hold the knee close to your chest until you can hold it for one minute. Do not increase the repetitions, only the length of time you hold the position. (Turn on your favorite music or program to listen to while doing this exercise.)

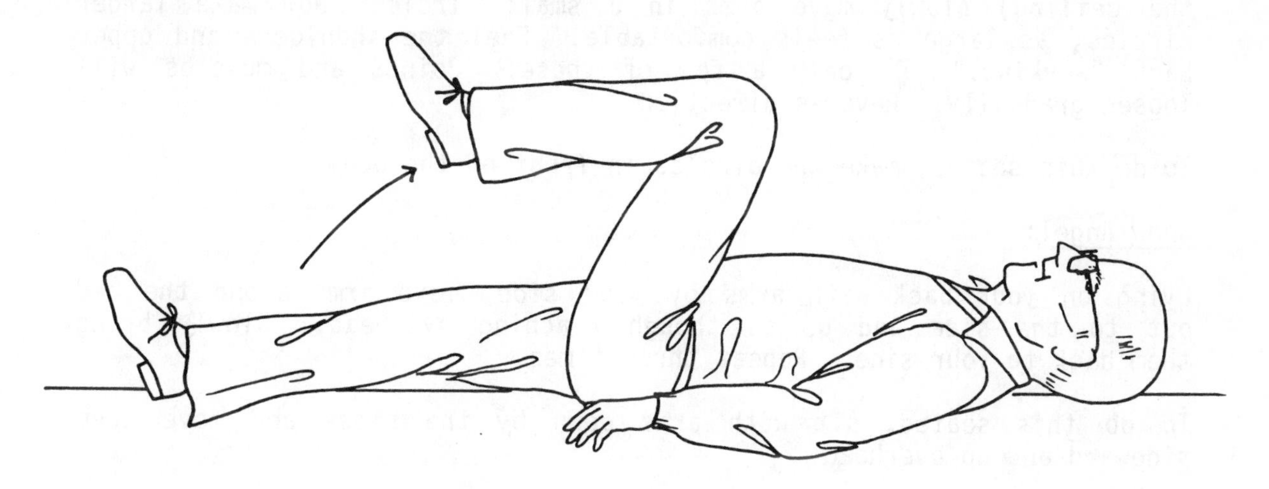

The knee lifts can be done while seated by bringing one knee at a time toward the chest and holding it there.

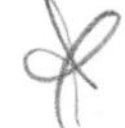

Both Knees to Chest (not recommended for persons with hip replacement):

Now bring both knees toward your chest and gently hold them there with your hands for 15 seconds. Lower your feet to the bed. Keep breathing while doing this. The next time you do this exercise, hold your knees a little longer until you work up to holding them there for 1 minute.

The following exercises are to keep upper body joints mobile and muscles stretched out. Check to make sure there is space to reach arms overhead.

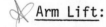

Arm Lift:

On your back, with the arms extended upward toward the ceiling, hold a rolled paper or hand towel with both hands so that arms are about shoulder width apart. Slowly, move arms with the elbows straight to the bed above your head. Now slowly bring them back to the ceiling still keeping the elbows straight. Maintain normal breathing during this stretching exercise. Try to relax rather than strain while doing this. Do one or two to begin with; just do what feels good. Flexibility is being emphasized.

To do this seated, hold arms out to the front at shoulder level, lift them up as far as is comfortable, and return to front.

Arm Circles:

Starting in the same position as the above exercise (holding the towel or paper roll with both hands elbows straight and arms pointing toward the ceiling) slowly move arms in a small circle. Now make larger circles, as large as feels comfortable. Feel the shoulders and upper back "working." Do only a few of these. Joints and muscles will loosen gradually. Reverse direction.

To do this seated, make the circles in front of the body.

Snow Angel:

Lying on your back with arms by your side, move arms along the bed out to the side and up as though reaching overhead. Slowly bring them back to your side. Repeat three times.

To do this seated, sit with arms down by the sides and move them sideward and up overhead.

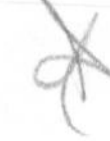

Arm Rolls:

To achieve the proper shoulder position, lie on your back with one arm straight out from the shoulder and resting on the bed. Now bend the elbow until the fingers point toward the ceiling. Begin the exercise by slowly lowering the hand to the bed by your hip, palm down. Return until fingers point toward the ceiling and continue until the back of the hand rests on the bed by your head. Return your hand to your hip. Repeat three times with each arm.

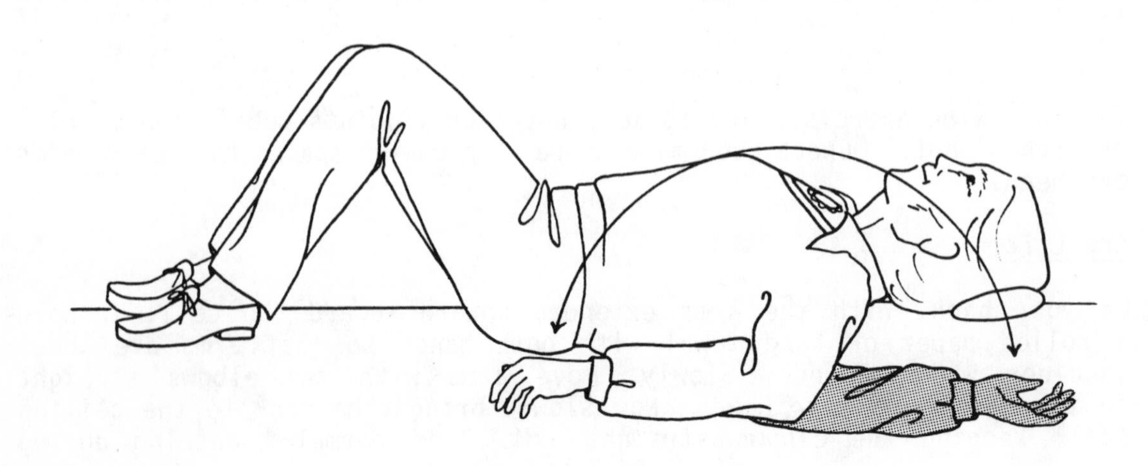

Session wrap-up; enjoy a snack if desired.

ENDING THE SESSION:

Share the basket.

Talk about and confirm next session.

AFTER THE SESSION:

Write up comments.

IDEAS FOR MODIFYING THE ACTIVITY: If the elder and leader cannot create a lying position for this session, it is possible to learn the exercises from a seated position. These modifications are listed at the end of each exercise description.

TIPS FOR SAFETY: Never do any exercise that causes pain. If you experience pain, stop the activity. These are to be done slowly and carefully. In order to get the benefit of stretching and moving a joint through its entire range of motion, move even those limbs with limited range to the fullest extent possible. Note to individuals who have had a hip replacement: AVOID LIFTING THE THIGH ON THAT LIMB ANY CLOSER TO THE BODY THAN IT IS WHEN IN A NORMAL SITTING POSITION (thigh and trunk making a 90-degree or right angle to each other). See the session "Total hip exercises" for a series of exercises that are safe to do.

Be cautious about getting down on the floor. Some older persons have difficulty getting up from the floor. Review page 18 on how to get up from the floor during a session. Do not encourage the elder to get on the floor if he/she does not want to. If the elder wants to do this session from a floor position, ask if he/she has gotten down and up from the floor recently. If there is a response indicating a long time has passed since being on the floor, or if the elder is obese or very weak, don't allow floor work. The leader must be responsible for not creating a situation necessitating lifting the elder. Moving the session into the bedroom or using a couch is preferable.

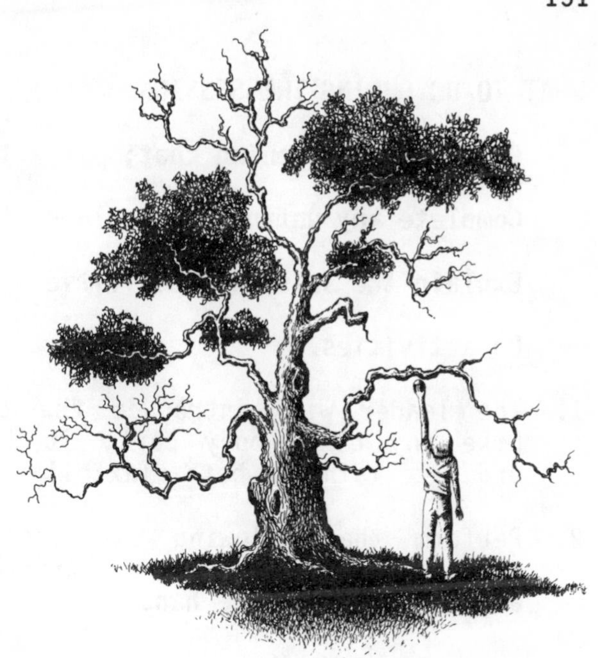

UNIT NAME: Exercises for Special Purposes

ACTIVITY PLAN 8: HAND/WRIST FLEXIBILITY AND STRENGTH

PURPOSE OF ACTIVITY: To focus on exercises that will keep hands flexible and strong and ease the pain caused by arthritis. These will help in performing daily activities that require grasping, turning, and twisting the hands.

DESCRIPTION OF ACTIVITY: The leader will explain the necessity of moving the joints to keep them flexible and will then perform the exercises, with the elder following along. A brief discussion will follow in which the leader and elder can share tips on care and protection of the hands.

BENEFITS OF ACTIVITY: This season provides simple, quick exercises that can be done at any time and place. Many people experience stiff, sore hands and need a reminder that a few minutes of attention to the hands can bring relief and prolong their strength and flexibility.

BEFORE THE SESSION:

Things to do

The leader should read through the activity plan to become familiar with the topic and today's exercises.

Things to take

Bring two foam balls. They should be about the size of a tennis ball. Foam balls are excellent for this purpose, as well as small homemade bean bags. Also bring two sheets of paper.

WHAT TO DO DURING THE SESSION:

Greeting and opening chat; pay attention to any immediate needs.

Complete any unfinished business from previous session.

Explain the session's activities.

Do activities.

1. The leader will introduce the topic by discussing these points. Like any other body part, it is important to USE the hands in order to maintain both flexibility and strength.

2. Perform the following exercises. Begin with three repetitions of each and increase to a comfortable level that produces a warming and limbering of the hands.

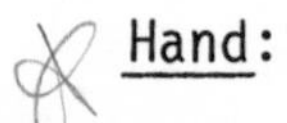

Hand:

Make a fist. Straighten the fingers. Spread fingers apart, keeping them straight. Bring fingers back together. Repeat.

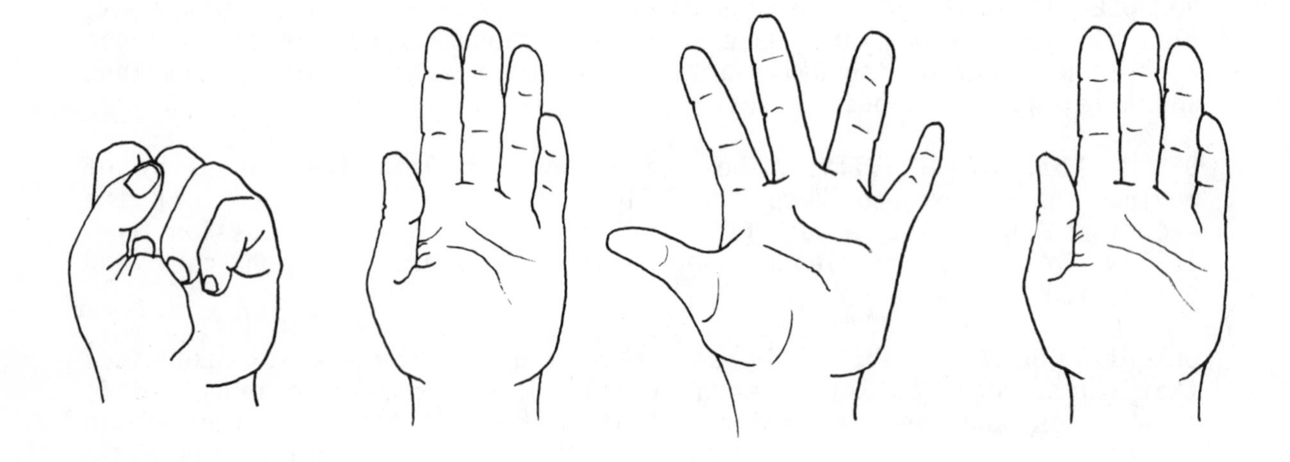

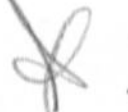

Thumb:

With hand open, place thumb across the palm of the hand. Bring thumb back out to the side away from the palm. Repeat. With palm up, fingers together, move thumb away from the palm. If you turn your hand sideways you have made an "L." Bring thumb back toward the palm. Repeat. Move thumb out to touch the tip of the little finger. Now touch the tip of each finger. Repeat, using each hand.

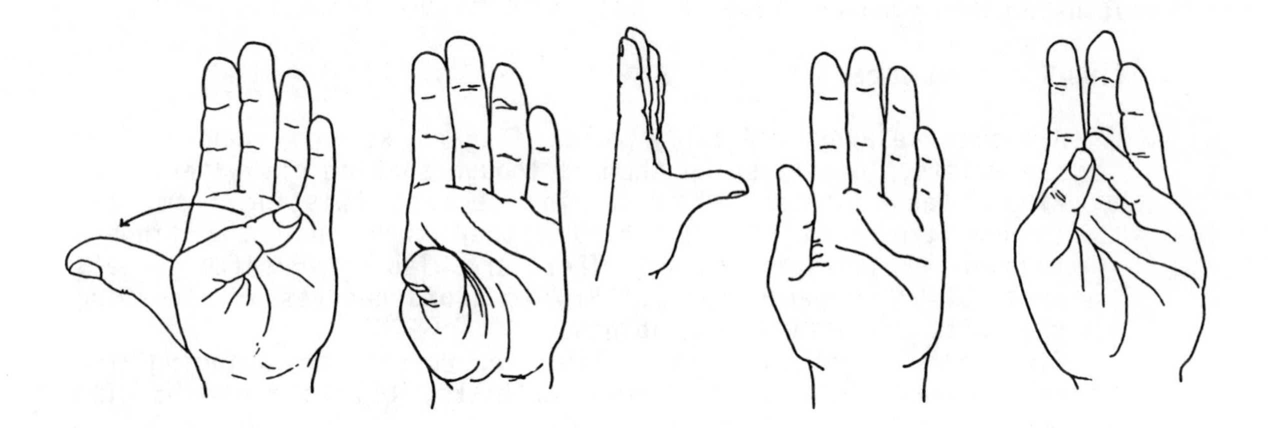

Wrist:

Bend wrists so that the palm is facing toward the forearm, fingers pointed toward the shoulders. Straighten wrist and move hand down so that palm is facing out. Repeat. Hold elbow up against side, palms down, and move wrist so that the thumb points toward the body. Move wrist in the other direction. As you go back and forth, left to right, you will be moving your hands like the windshield wipers on a car. Move wrists in circles. Circle in one direction and then the other.

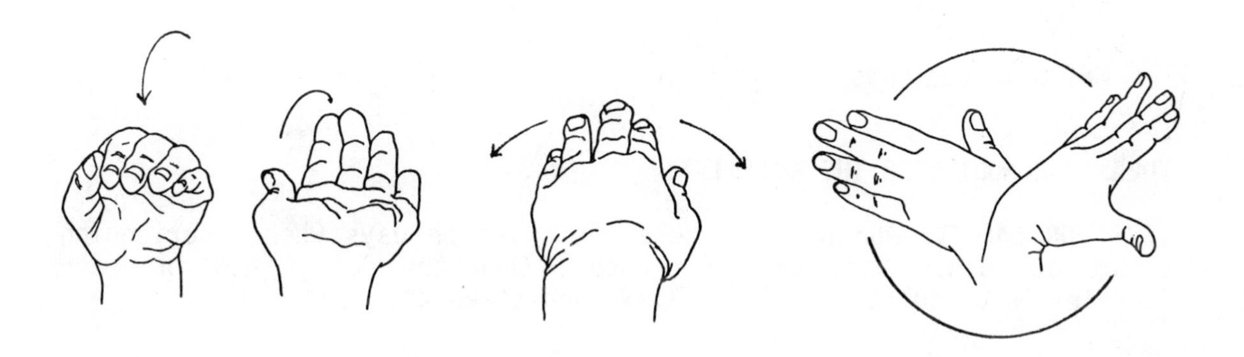

Grip:

Hold a soft, foam ball or bean bag in one hand and squeeze it; then transfer it to the other hand and squeeze it. Then roll the ball around between the palms and fingers of one hand. Roll between two hands.

In one hand hold a sheet of paper and try to crumple it into a ball. Now, still using one hand, slowly uncrumple the balled-up paper. Repeat using other hand.

3. Tips for hand care:

   a. All-over relaxer: Totally relax fingers so they dangle from the wrists. Gently shake them as though shaking off water.
   b. Fingers and joints: When opening jars by twisting them, try to use the palm of your hand rather than just the fingers to apply pressure and twist. There are also some useful gadgets available for opening jars. Try to avoid unnecessary twisting that puts a strain on the joints.
   c. Fingers and joints: When doing exercises or swinging the arms around while doing household tasks, try to avoid banging hands against furniture.
   d. Whole hand: Gentle massaging will warm the hands and ease stiffness. If hands are very painful, trade massages between elder and leader.

Session wrap-up; enjoy a snack if desired.

ENDING THE SESSION:

Share the basket.

Talk about and confirm next session.

AFTER THE SESSION:

Write up comments.

IDEAS FOR MODIFYING THE ACTIVITY:

TIPS FOR SAFETY: Do not do these exercises on days when experiencing a lot of pain. Once the pain eases, then try doing them in order to maintain circulation, flexibility, and strength.

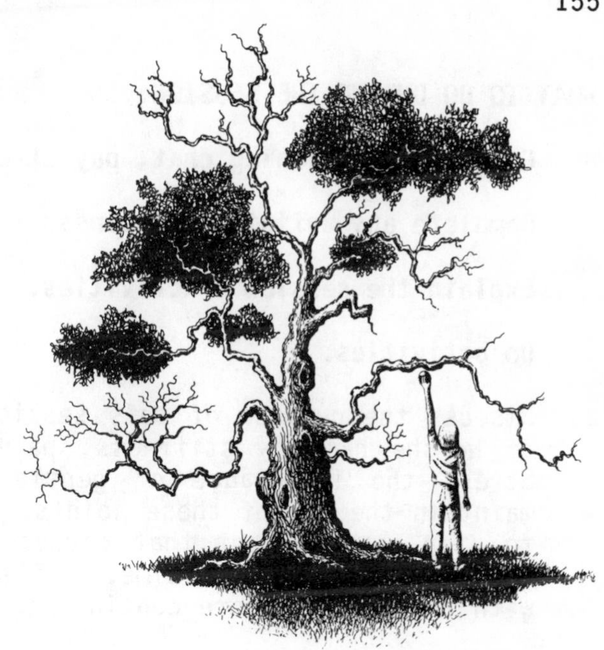

UNIT NAME: Exercises for Special Purposes

ACTIVITY PLAN 9: TOTAL HIP EXERCISES

PURPOSE OF ACTIVITY: To maintain mobility in hip joints. This is particularly useful for persons who have had hip surgery. The exercises increase mobility and build strength, endurance, and coordination.

DESCRIPTION OF ACTIVITY: The leader will go over this series of exercises with the elder, clarify directions, and go through them as the elder tries them out on a bed, couch, or the floor. With a copy of the exercises on hand, the elder may perform the exercises during the week; three times per week, skipping one day between exercises. Monday-Wednesday-Friday or Tuesday-Thursday-Saturday are typical patterns.

BENEFITS OF ACTIVITY: This series of exercises can be done in bed. They are beneficial for maintenance of strength and flexibility and coordination for everyone. For individuals who have had hip replacements, it is even more important to continue these exercises three times a week.

BEFORE THE SESSION:

Things to do

Things to take

WHAT TO DO DURING THE SESSION:

Greeting and opening chat; pay attention to any immediate needs.

Complete any unfinished business from previous session.

Explain the session's activities.

Do activities.

1. Discuss the purpose of this session with the elder. Ask the elder if he/she has any stiffness, pain or limited motion in the hips. Stress the importance of gentle, careful movement of joints to maintain the use of these joints. Stress also that it is important to stop any movement that causes pain. If the pain is temporary, try again at another time. If pain doesn't go away, discuss it with the doctor before continuing. Do the following exercises:

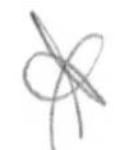

Hip Flexion:

Lie on your back and raise one knee toward but not all the way to the chest. Keep lower leg, or calf, parallel to the bed so that the thigh and bed form a right angle. Lower the leg to the bed, straightening it. Repeat. Begin with 3 repetitions with each leg and slowly increase to 10 to 15 with each leg.

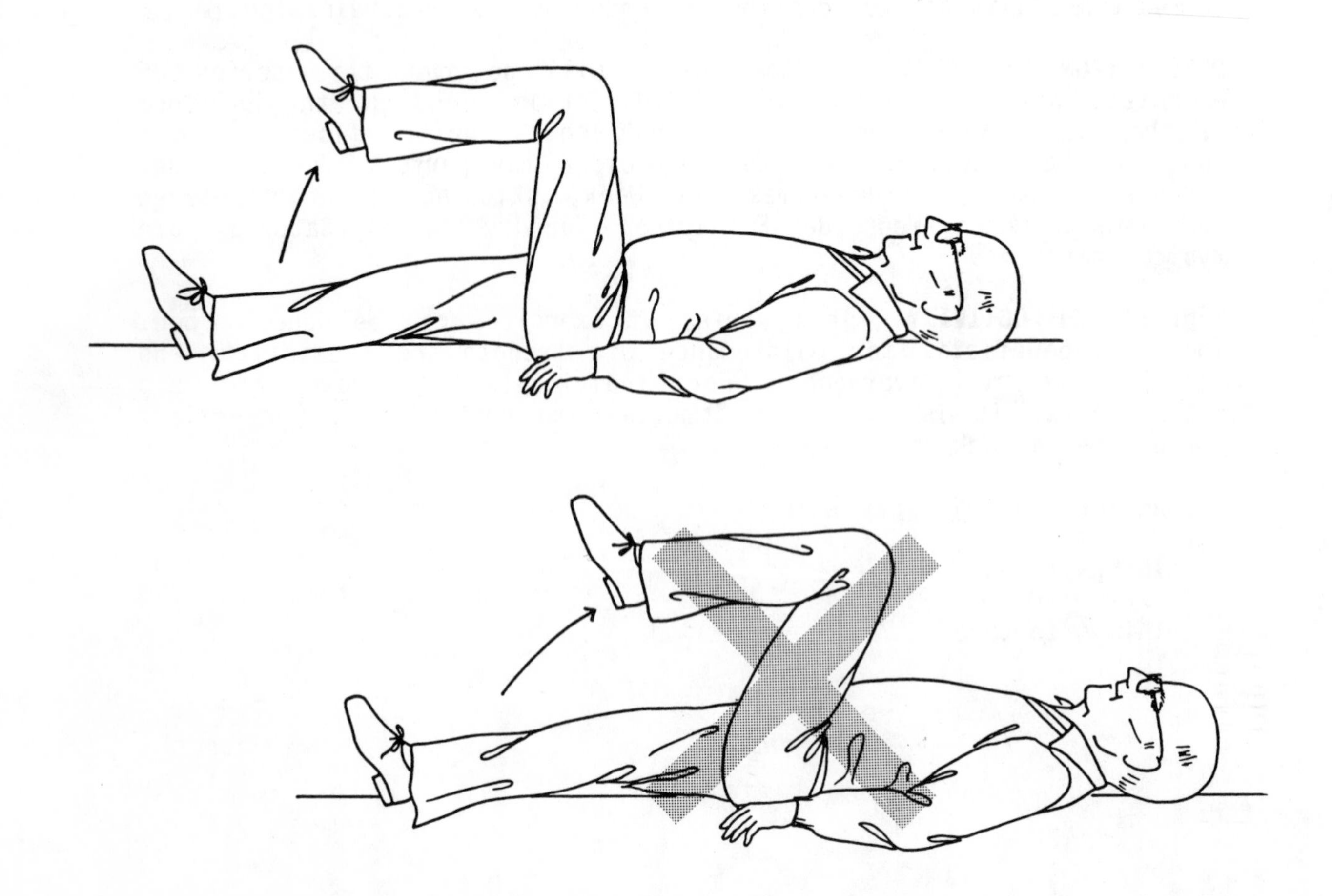

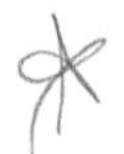

Straight Leg Raises:

Lie on your back, bend one hip and knee; the foot is flat on the mat. This will help keep your back flat during the exercise to protect it from strain. Keeping the other leg straight, lift it from the mat approximately 6 inches, hold for 5 seconds, then lower it to the mat, rest 10 seconds. Repeat. Begin with 3 repetitions per leg and increase gradually to 10 to 15.

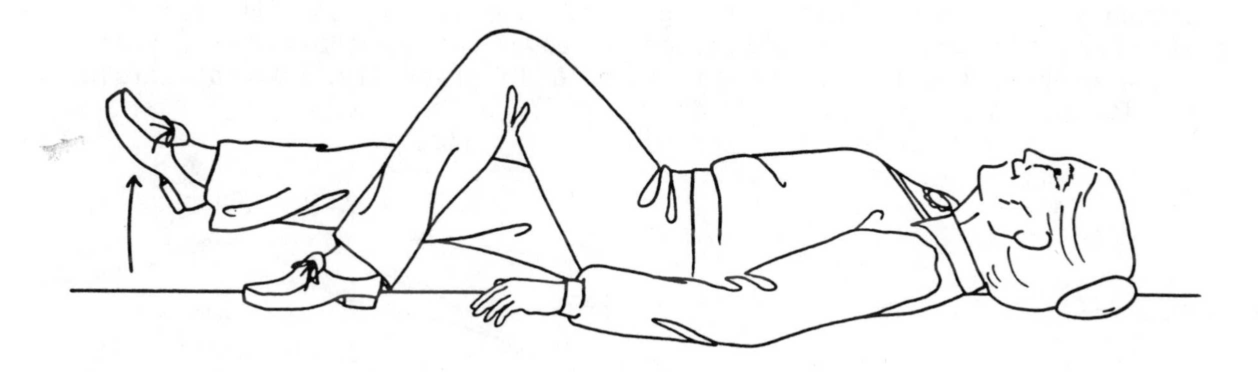

Hip Abduction: (leg to side)

Lie on your back (or stand behind a chair) with your body in good alignment. Keep leg on the bed. Slide the leg out to the side as far as possible. Be sure to keep leg straight and DO NOT bend at the waist. Return leg to the middle so that it rests next to the other leg. Repeat. Begin with 3 repetitions per leg, and gradually increase to 10 to 15 times.

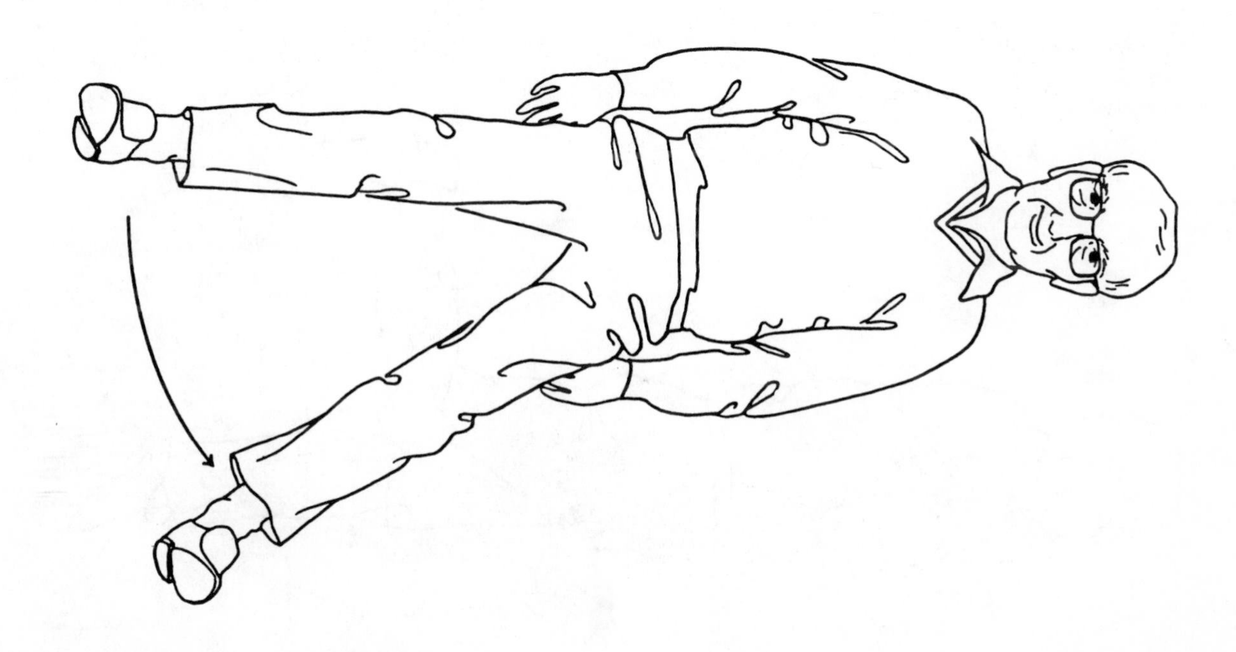

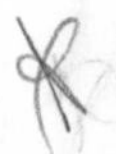

Gluteal Exercises:

Lie on your back; squeeze buttocks together firmly. Hold for three to five counts, relax, and repeat. Do not hold your breath! Continue to breathe normally even when you squeeze. Begin with 3 repetitions and increase to 10 to 15.

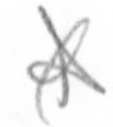

Hip Extension 1:

Lie on your stomach. Raise one leg up off the mat, keeping it straight. It will come up only a few inches. Lower it to the mat. Repeat. Begin with 3 repetitions and increase to 10 gradually. Do not strain the lower back.

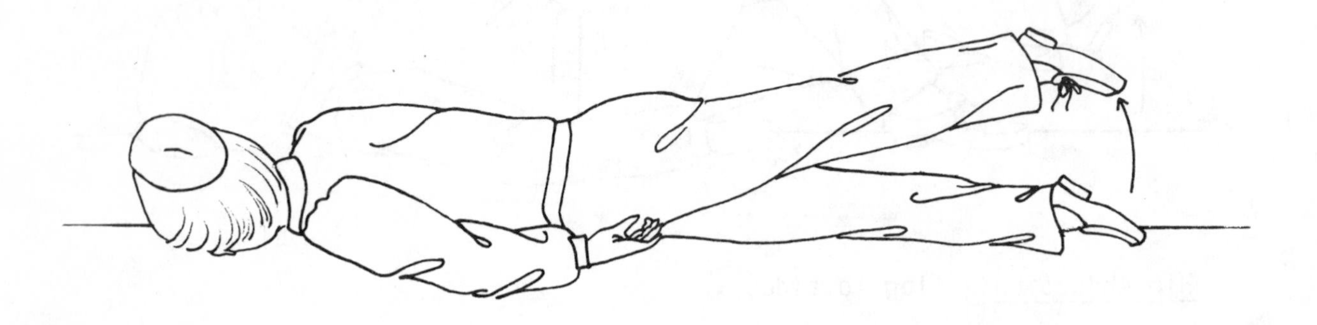

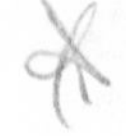

Hip Extension 2:

Lie on your stomach. Bend one knee so that the foot is toward the ceiling; then raise knee up slightly off the mat. Straighten leg by lowering foot back to the mat. Bend knee and repeat the process. Begin with 3 repetitions per leg and gradually increase to 10.

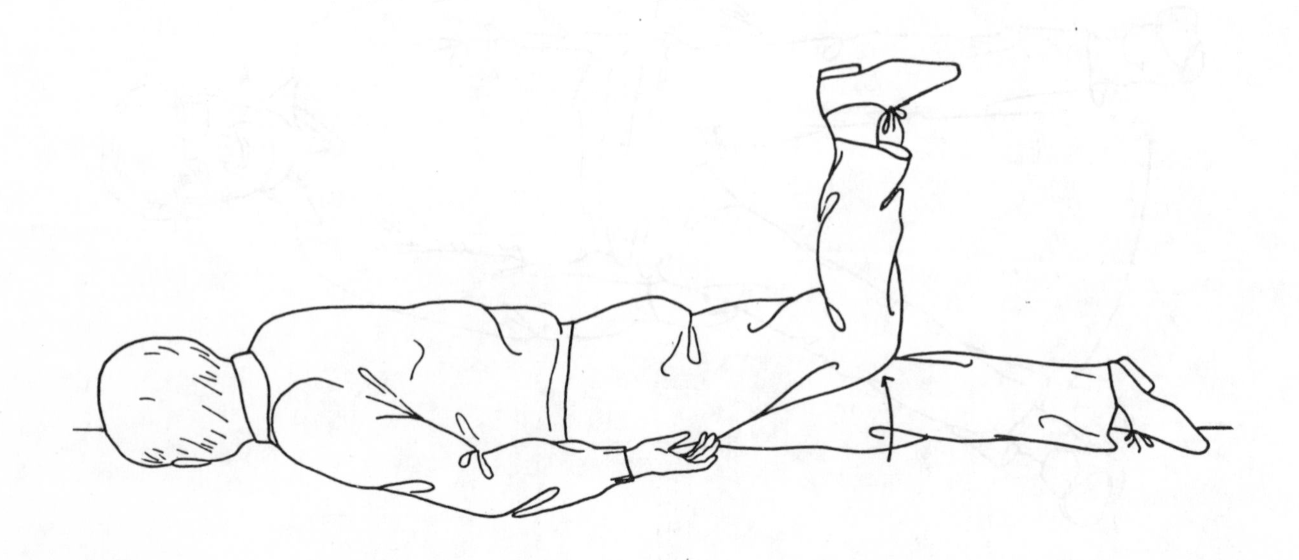

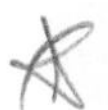

Standing Hip Flexion:

Stand and support yourself by holding onto a countertip, chair back, or table with one hand. Raise one knee up only to hip level; hold for 4 seconds. Return leg to standing position. Repeat. Begin with 3 repetitions per leg and increase to 10.

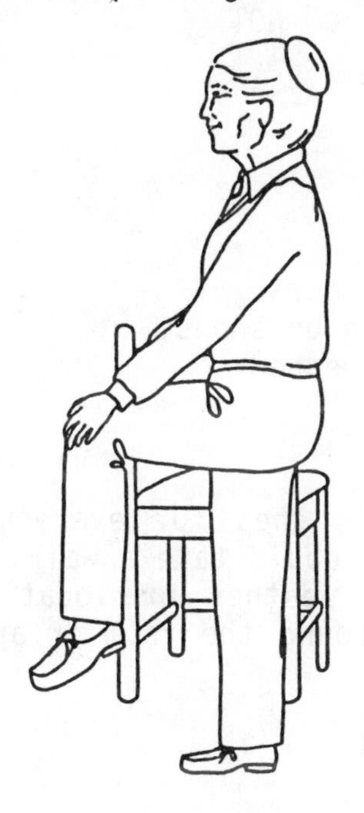

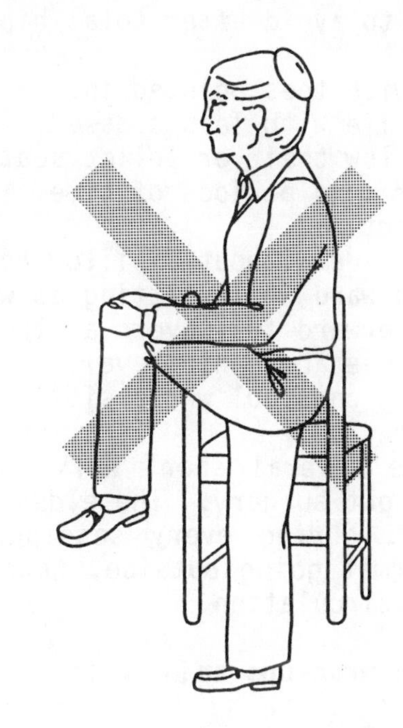

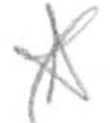

Standing Hip Extension:

Stand and hold onto a support for balance. Extend one leg backward slowly; keep it straight; hold it for 4 seconds. Do not bend forward. Repeat. Begin with 3 repetitions per leg. Gradually increase to 10.

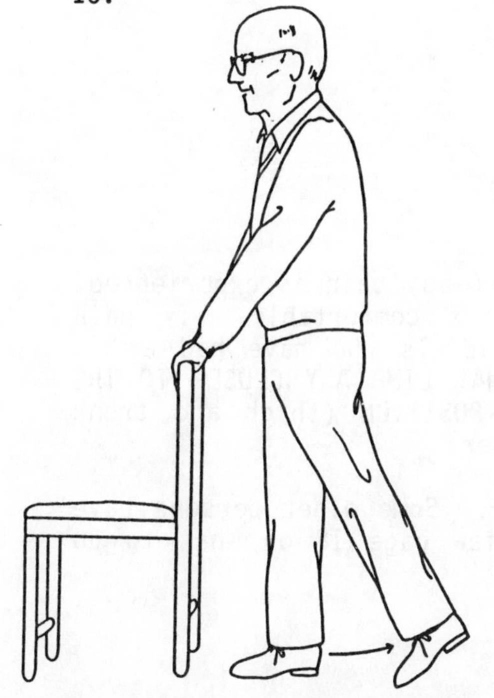

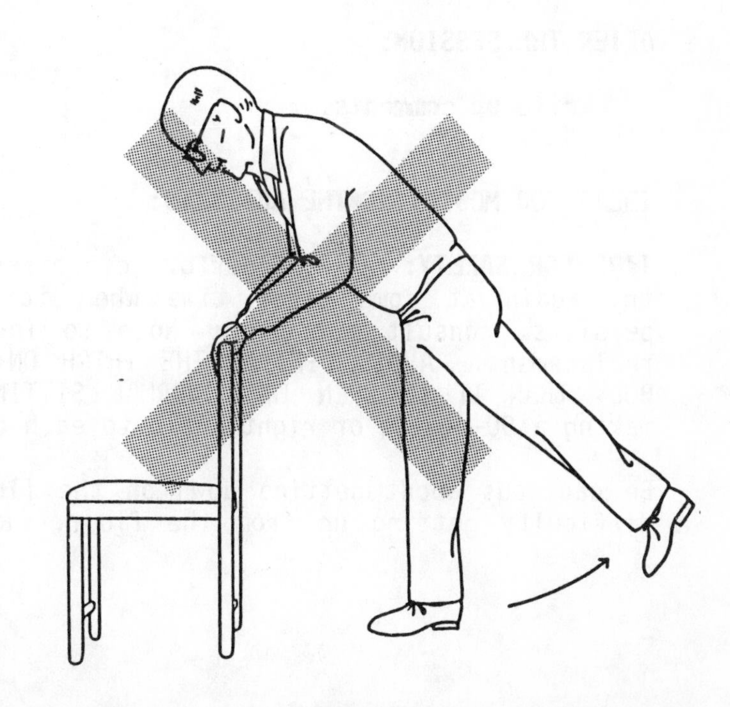

2. Explain that these are to be done every other day or three times a week with a day of rest between each session. Point out that these exercises build strength in the muscles that support the hip joints, as well as keep them flexible to maintain the ability to walk, sit, and rise.

3. Things to avoid after total hip surgery. DO NOT:

   Stand with toes pointed in.
   Sit or lie with legs crossed.
   Sit on low chair or toilet seat.
   Sit for long periods of time.
   Get overtired.
   Lie on side without a pillow between the knees.
   Lean forward while sitting as when putting on shoes.
   Reach forward for covers at the foot of the bed.
   Raise knee above hip level.
   Put foot on stool while sitting.

4. DO take several short walks daily. This goes for everyone, with or without surgery. The elder and leader could take a walk, indoors or out, during every session. If the weather or location does not permit going outside, take a walk around the room or apartment to aid circulation.

   Session wrap-up; enjoy a snack if desired.

ENDING THE SESSION:

Share the basket.

Talk about and confirm next session.

AFTER THE SESSION:

Write up comments.

IDEAS FOR MODIFYING THE ACTIVITY:

TIPS FOR SAFETY: Do not perform exercises if any pain is experienced; try again at some other time when it feels comfortable. If pain persists, consult a doctor. Note to individuals who have had a hip replacement: AVOID LIFTING THE THIGH ON THAT LIMB ANY CLOSER TO THE BODY THAN IT IS WHEN IN A NORMAL SITTING POSITION (thigh and trunk making a 90-degree or right angle to each other).

Be cautious about getting down on the floor. Some older persons have difficulty getting up from the floor. Review page 18 on what to do if the elder falls or is found lying on the floor during a session. Do not encourage the elder to get on the floor. If the elder wants to do this session from a floor position, ask if he/she has gotten down and up from the floor recently. If there is a response indicating a long time has passed since being on the floor, or if the elder is obese or very weak, do not allow floor work. The leader must be responsible for not creating a situation necessitating lifting the elder. Moving the session into the bedroom or using a couch is preferable.

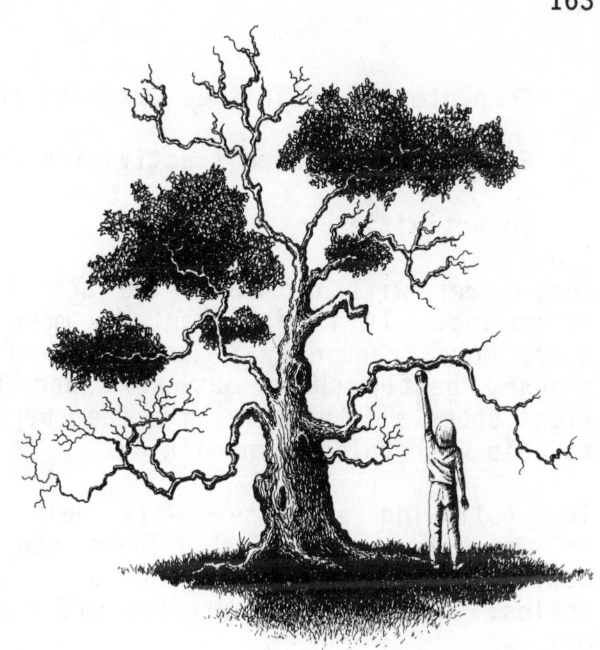

UNIT NAME: Exercises for Special Purposes

ACTIVITY PLAN 10: FEET AND ANKLE EXERCISES FOR BALANCE, STRENGTH, AND FLEXIBILITY

PURPOSE OF ACTIVITY: To discuss the importance of moving to maintain flexibility and strength. To present a series of feet and ankle exercises helping to maintain function in the feet.

BENEFITS OF ACTIVITY: These exercises are simple to follow and easy to do; they quickly become favorite exercises to do all through the day.

BEFORE THE SESSION:

Things to do

The leader should read through the activity plan to become familiar with the topic and exercises.

Things to take

Bring two foam balls and something shaped like a cylinder, such as an old rolling pin, a plastic bottle, or a can of food, which can safely be used to roll on the floor.

WHAT TO DO DURING THE SESSION:

Greeting and opening chat; pay attention to any immediate needs.

Complete any unfinished business from previous session.

Explain the session's activities.

Do activities.

The leader will introduce the activities by stressing the importance of moving. It is important to move the entire body at least every hour, more frequently if possible. Change positions, get up and walk around, gently shake out arms and legs. When they are encased in tight shoes all the time, the feet become stiff and cannot work properly to help with balance in walking.

The following exercises will help regain strength and flexibility in the feet and ankles. These can be done anywhere, anytime. The action of exercising will also prevent or lessen swollen feet and ankles. Seated foot exercises are most effective when done with shoes off.

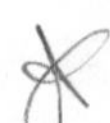

Foot Circling:

Lift one foot off the floor and trace a circle in the air with the toes. Make the circle as large as possible. Do three circles clockwise and three counterclockwise. Repeat using the other foot.

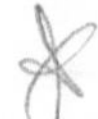

Windshield Washers:

Begin with feet flat on the floor, side by side. Keeping heels in place, slide toes as far as possible to the right and then to the left. Repeat this motion for a count of 16, one count per side.

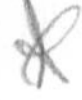

Toe-Heel:

Keeping heels on the floor, lift toes as high as possible. Put toes back down and lift the heels as high as possible. Repeat five times, moving one foot at a time or both feet together.

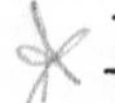

Toe Curls:

Curl toes under, toward the ball of the foot; then curl toes upward, toward the knees. Repeat five times.

Toe Spreads:

Spread your toes apart. Pull them back together. Wiggle them around, trying to spread them as much as possible. This may be hard at first, but you can "train" them to respond.

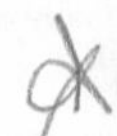

Step on a Ball:

Assume a forward stride position with one foot forward, the other foot nearer the chair. Place a foam ball under the forward foot and step on it until the ball is flattened. Repeat five times. Change foot positions and repeat with other foot five times.

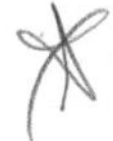
Foot Massage:

Place an old rolling pin, a sturdy plastic bottle, or can of food on the floor and roll it back and forth with your foot, "massaging" your entire foot from heel to toe.

Session wrap-up; enjoy a snack if desired.

ENDING THE SESSION:

Share the basket.

Talk about and confirm next session.

AFTER THE SESSION:

Write up comments.

IDEAS FOR MODIFYING THE ACTIVITY: Sharing a foot massage or massaging one's own feet would be nice. If the elder and leader care to do this, they should bathe the feet before the session. If the floor is not carpeted, spread a small towel on the floor and try to wrinkle it with the toes.

TIPS FOR SAFETY: These exercises should be done seated in a sturdy chair. As cautioned in all exercises, stop if there is any pain and discontinue the particular movement that causes pain until a doctor's comments can be obtained. Do exercises that are comfortable in order to maintain use of those parts of the body.

REFERENCES AND RESOURCES

Bender, R. Yoga exercises for every body. Avon, CT: Ruben Publishing, 1975.

Fifty positive vigor exercises for senior citizens. Reston, VA: American Alliance of Health, Physical Education, Recreation and Dance Publications, Physical Education Recreation for the Handicapped, Information and Utilization Center, 1981.

Home program exercises: Total hip, back, shoulders and arms, hands, feet. Ames, IA: Mary Greeley Medical Center, Physical Therapy Department, 1982.

Noble, E. Essential exercises for the childbearing years. Boston: Houghton Mifflin, 1976.

Washburn, B. K., & Swanson, M. A. Neck care. Redmond, WA: Medic Publishing Company, 1979.

APPENDICES

APPENDIX A
Audiovisuals

Slides that depict vision changes in the aged:

Vision Kit
Dr. Leon Postalan
The Gerontology Center
University of Michigan
Ann Arbor, Michigan 48109

(Dr. Postalan's slides are accompanied by a script.)

Vision Kit
Dr. Gary Ross
Gerontology Program
University of Nebraska at Omaha
Omaha, Nebraska 68132

(Dr. Ross's slides have a tape that can be played on a cassette tape recorder to accompany the slides.)

Goggles that change the inclination of the floor and depict visual difficulties encountered in walking may be obtained from:

Goggles Kit
Pentagon Services Corporation
21 Harriet Drive
Syosset, New York 11791

Tapes that depict hearing changes as a person gets older:

Hearing Tape
Dr. Gary Ross
Gerontology Program
University of Nebraska at Omaha
Omaha, Nebraska 68132

Getting Through (Record)
1970 Zenith Corporation
6501 West Grand Avenue
Chicago, Illinois 60635

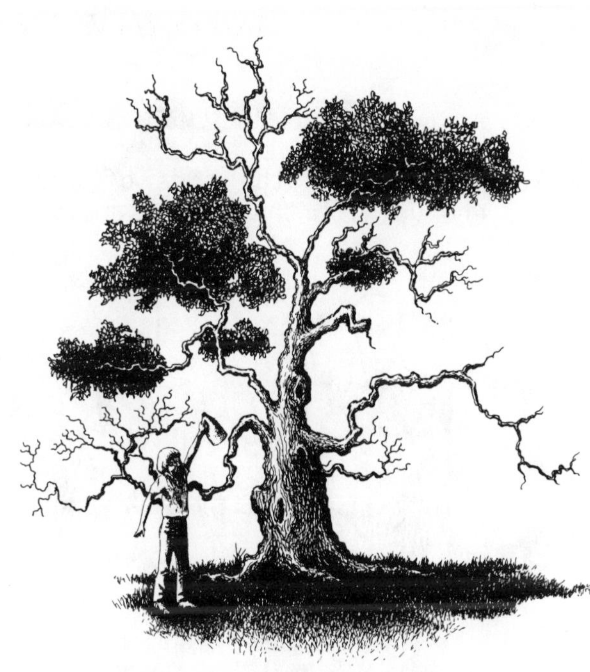

APPENDIX B

Exercises for Strength: Illustrations and Exercises Charts

This appendix contains illustrations of each exercise and an exercise chart to record progress.

The bar code following the name of each exercise indicates for which activity plan that exercise is used. For example, if an exercise is used in ACTIVITY PLANS 4, 5, 6, 7, 8, 9, 10, then all boxes except 4 through 10 are darkened, as illustrated.

■	4	5	6	7	8	9	10

As the sessions progress, the number of repetitions for each exercise is increased, and the resistance or weight lifted increases. This is consistent with the overload principle of muscular strength development. Do only those exercises approved by the physician. If all are approved, try to do as many as possible. There will be days when it is not possible to do some of the exercises due to pain or other illness. At these times it is best to rest until another time.

1. TOAST YOUR ARMS

3 6 9

Sitting upright in the chair, hold one hand at the side of your chair. Raise your arm slowly forward and up with the elbow straight and return slowly.

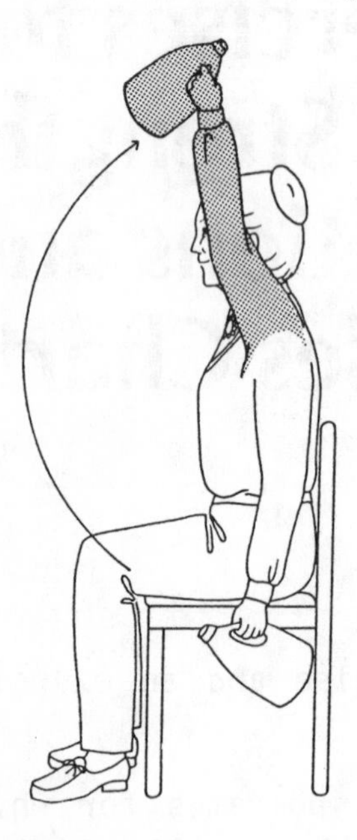

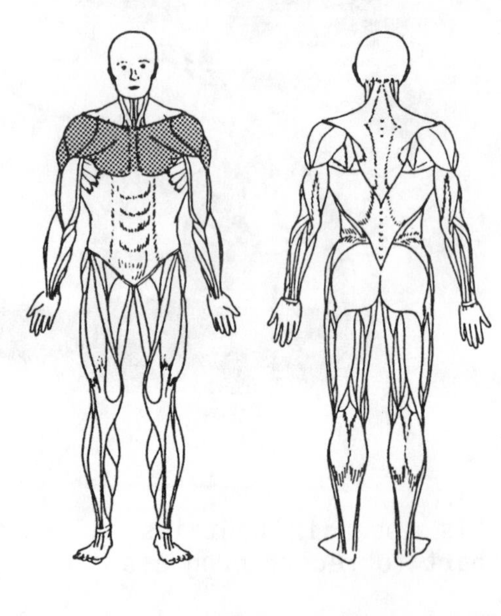

2. TAKE A LITTLE DRINK

3 6 9

Sitting upright in the chair, hold one hand at the side of your chair. Raise your forearms slowly forward and up with the elbow straight and return slowly.

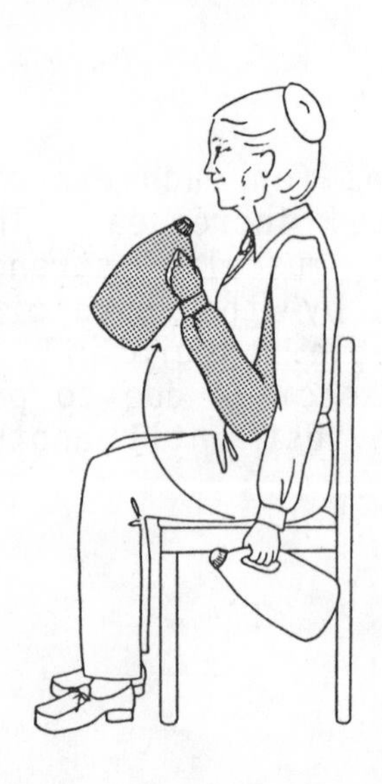

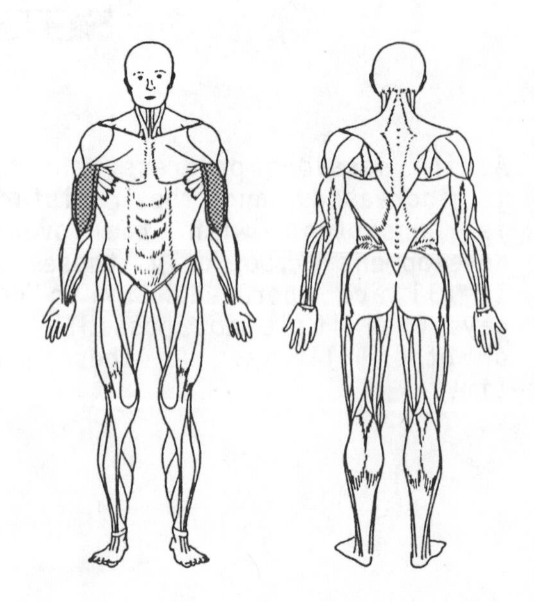

3. SWING A GARDEN GATE

4 6 9

Sitting in a chair, hold your plastic bottles in front of your chest and gently rock it left and right. Make the hinge for your gate be your wrist while the rest of your arm stays motionless. Sing a children's song as you swing your gate first in your left hand and then in your right hand.

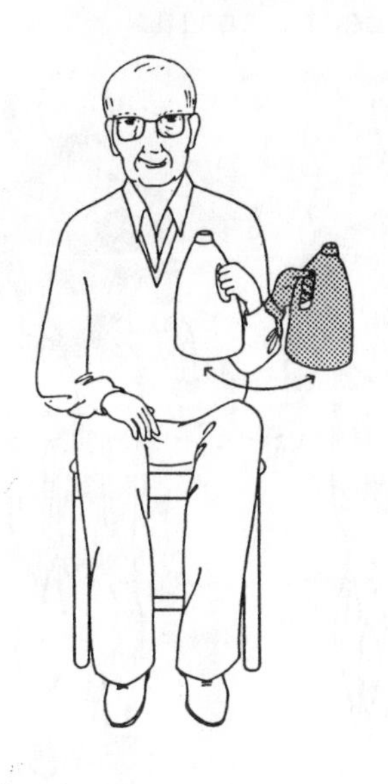

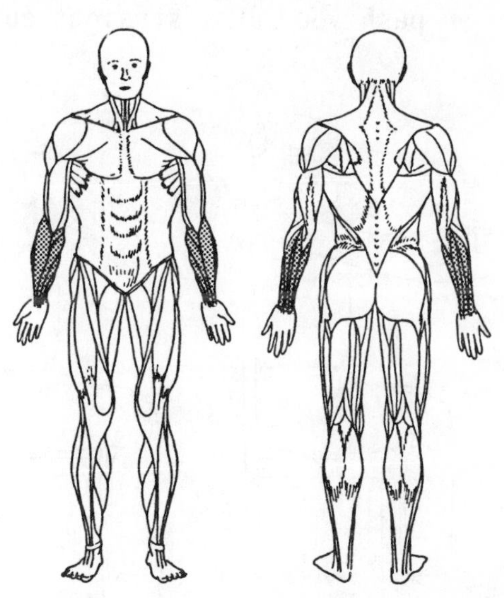

4. SITTING JACKS

4 6 9

Sit with your best sitting posture and your arms hanging to your sides. Raise your arms straight to the side toward the ceiling. Can you touch your hands over your head? Return your arms on the same path and repeat the lift slowly.

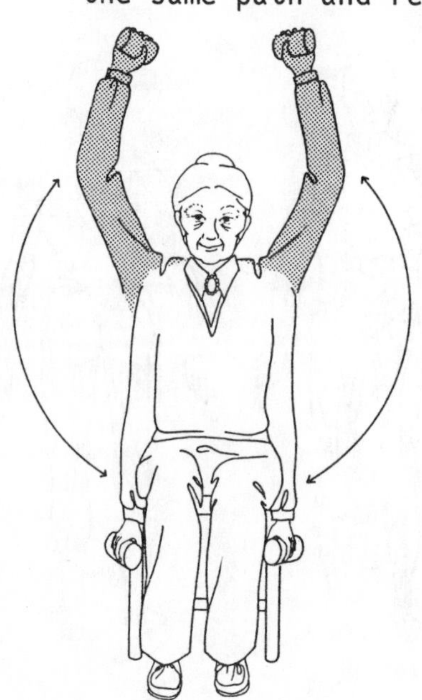

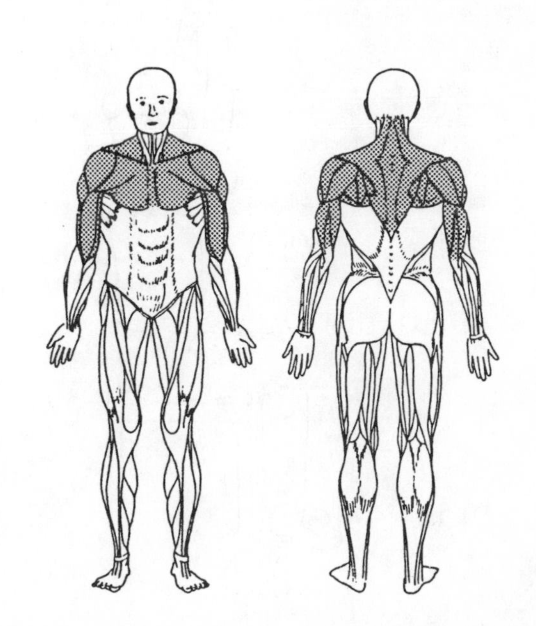

5. SWIM THE BREAST STROKE

3 8 10

Sitting upright in the chair, reach both arms out straight in front of your chest, hands touching. Pull your arms apart to your sides, keeping them at shoulder level; don't allow them to drop to your sides. Once you've pulled your arms apart to your sides, bend your elbows and bring your hands to your chest. Then push your arms straight out in front of you and begin again.

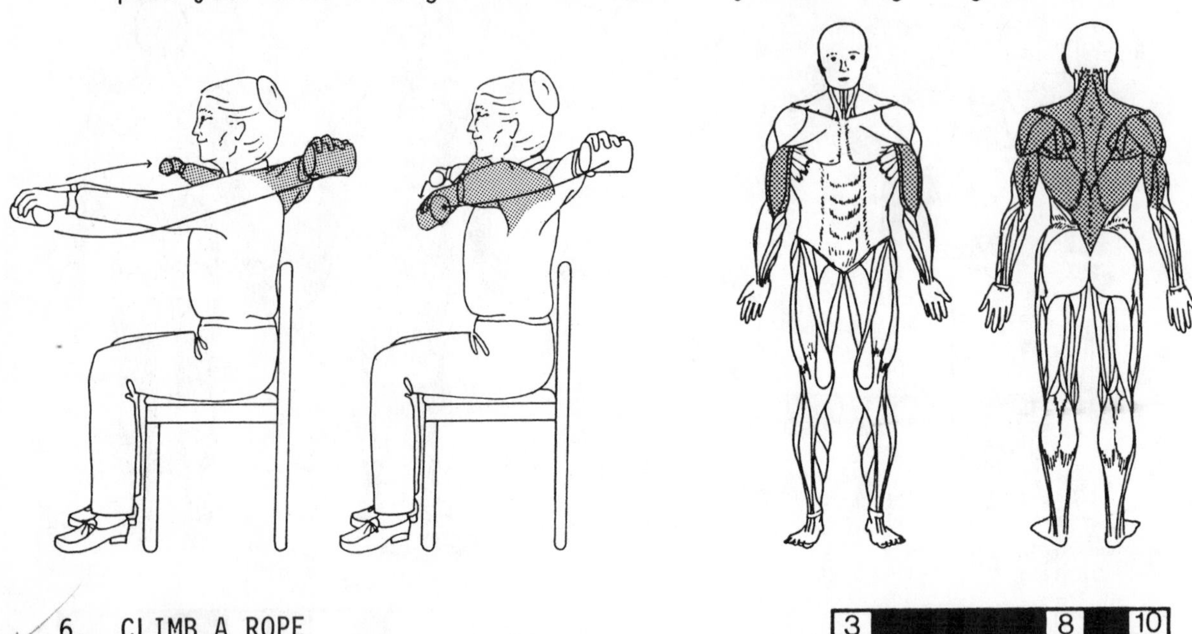

6. CLIMB A ROPE

3 8 10

Sitting in a chair, raise both arms overhead. Alternately bend elbows and lower each hand in front of your face and return it overhead. Lower right, lower left, reach up right, reach up left, and continue.

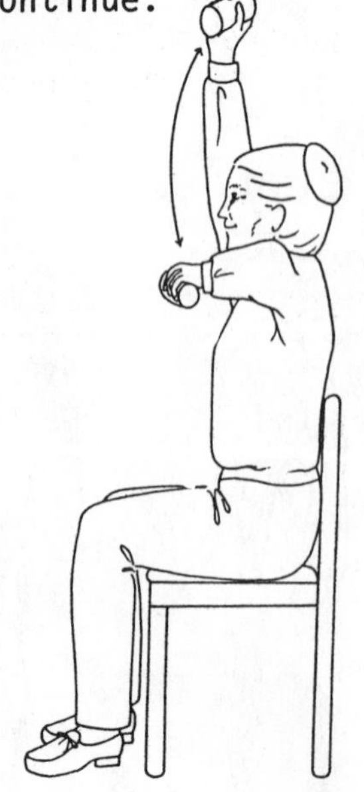

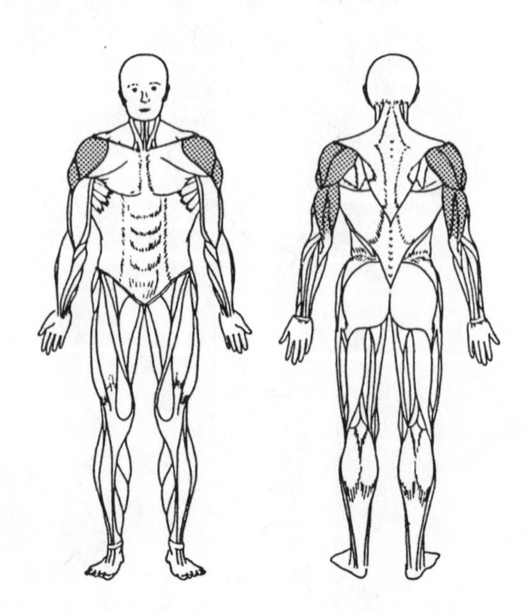

7. TAKE OFF YOUR HAT

4 8 10

Sitting in a chair, raise both arms overhead and then bend one elbow and lower the hand behind your head. Raise it back upward to join the other hand. Now bend your other elbow and lower the hand behind your head. Raise it back upward to join the other hand.

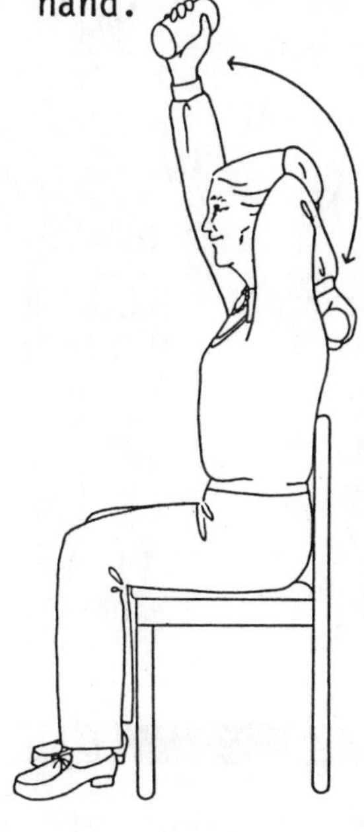

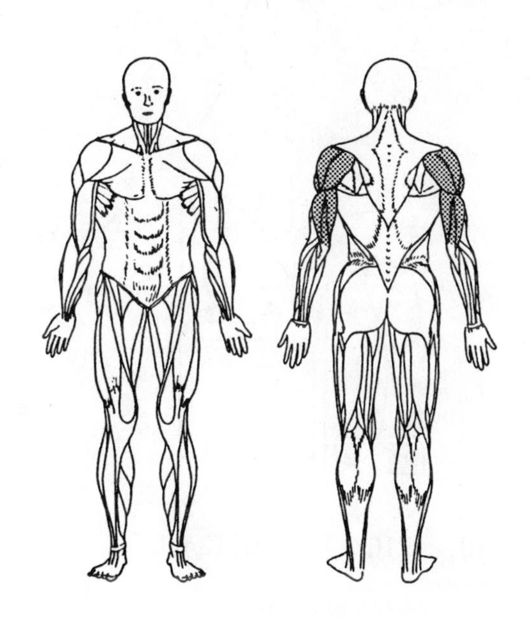

8. WALK A TIGHTROPE

4 8 10

When a tightrope walker starts to fall backward, he/she circles both arms to regain balance. You can do this same motion slowly without even fearing a fall! Sitting straight and tall, let your arms hang to the sides of your chair. Moving both arms forward, make large circles forward-up-back-down; forward-up-back-down.

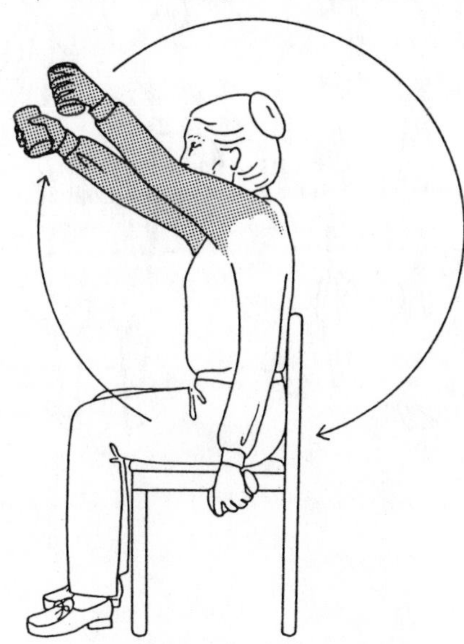

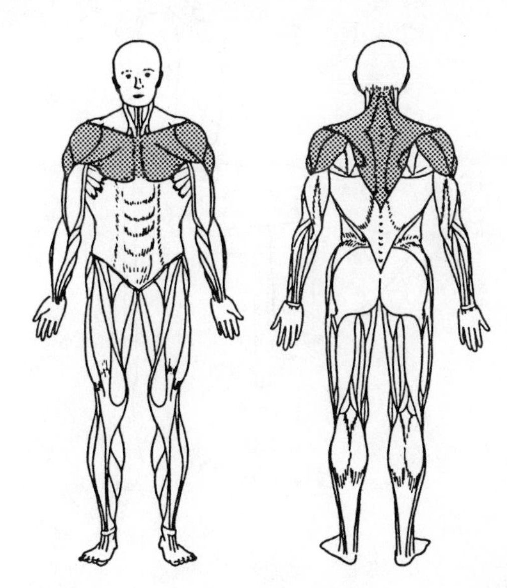

9. MARCH A MILE

3 6 9

Sitting upright in the chair, begin by lifting one knee and then the other. Don't lift too high or too fast.

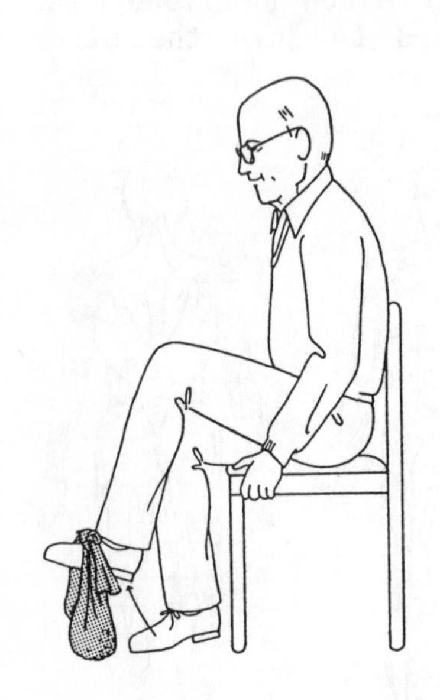

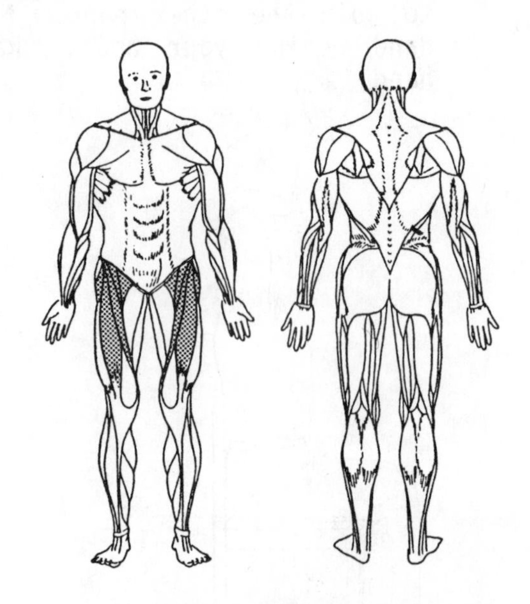

10. KICK THE FOOTBALL

4 8 9

Sitting in a chair, straighten your leg out in front of your chair. Bend your knee and return the foot to the floor. Do this lift slowly with one leg, then repeat with the other.

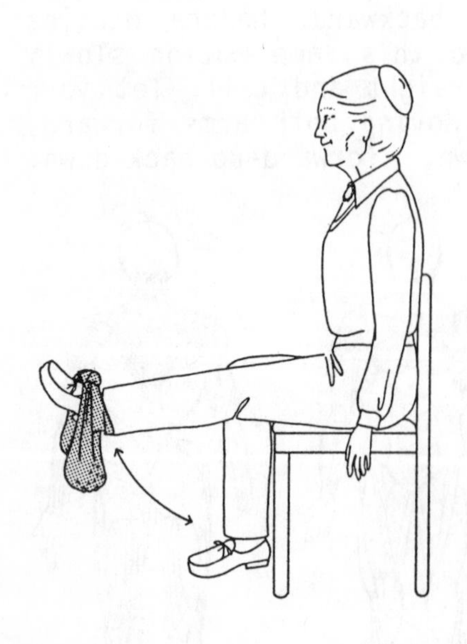

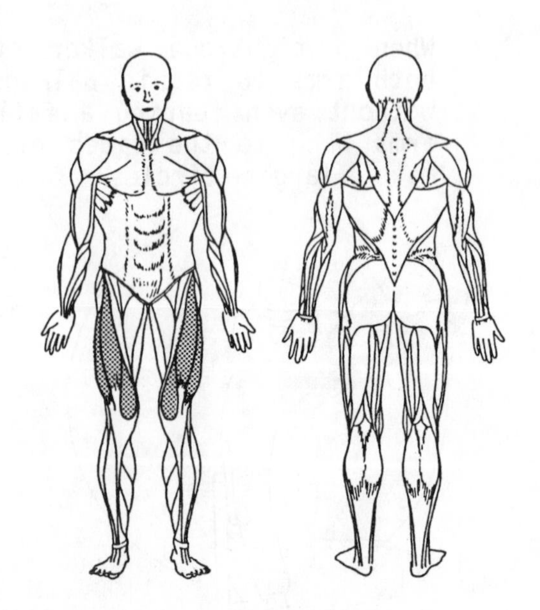

11. RAISE YOUR TOES

4 6 9

Sit in a chair with your legs crossed if possible; if not, support your leg off the ground by clasping your knee in interlocked fingers and lean back as shown in the exercise illustration. Using just your ankle, raise your toes slightly.

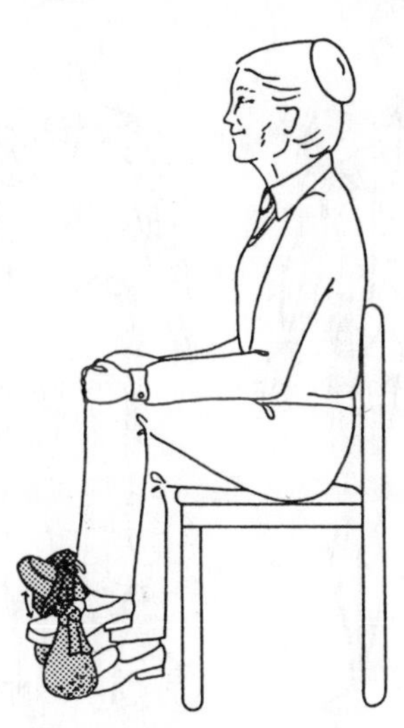

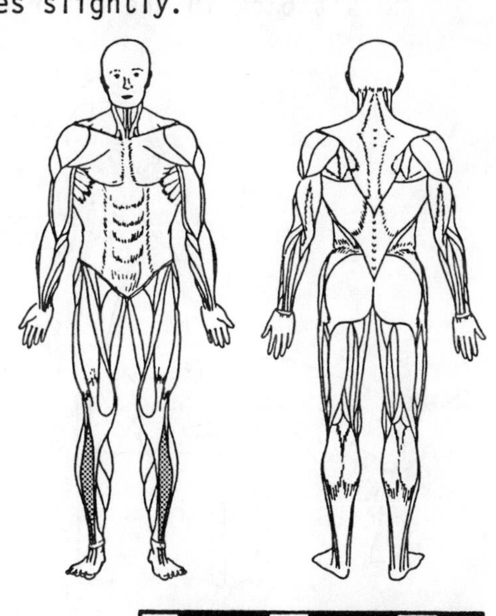

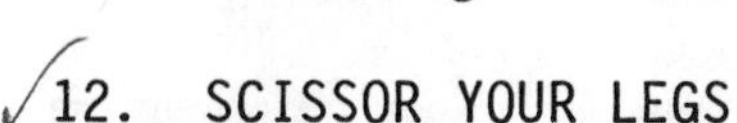

12. SCISSOR YOUR LEGS

3 6 9

Sitting in a chair, stretch your legs out on the floor in front of you. Raise your feet off the floor and spread your legs apart. Keeping your feet off the floor, bring your legs together and then lower your legs and rest. This exercise is strenuous and should not be repeated without a rest. Two or three repetitions should be enough. Be sure to sit back in the chair and not arch your lower back in this exercise.

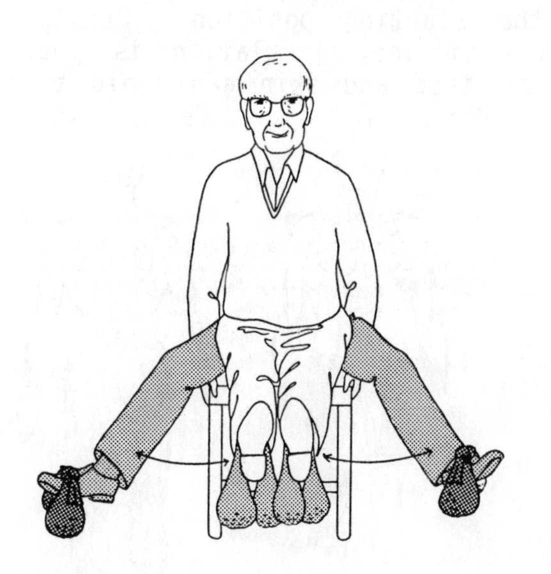

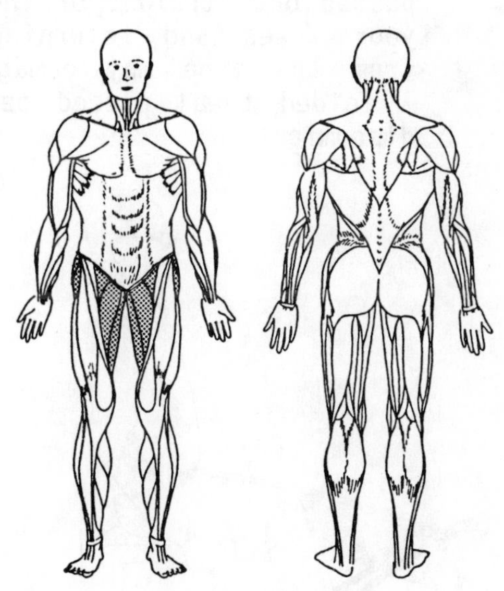

13. FLUTTER KICK

3 6 9

Sitting in a chair, stretch your legs out on the floor in front of you. Raise one foot and then another off the floor slowly. Keep these alternate lifts going for two more times. Be sure to sit back in the chair and don't arch your lower back.

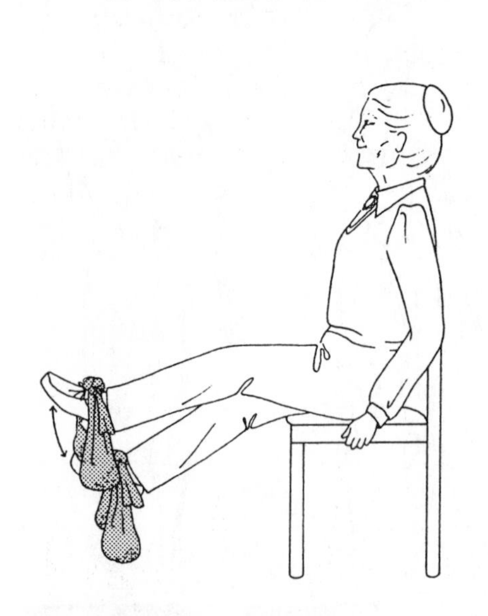

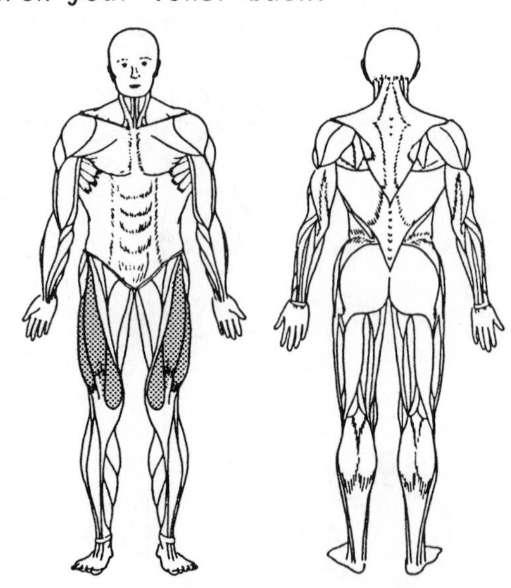

14. THE BEAR TRAP

5 7 10

Hook the inner tube under the front legs of your chair as shown in the exercise illustration. This is nearly impossible to do while sitting in the chair! Once the tube is in position sit upright in the chair and slip both your feet into the loop. Now you are trapped! Push forward with your legs and feel the tube pressing on the tops of your ankles. When your legs are pushed out straight or the tube is stretched tight, begin bending your knees and returning to the starting position. Pressure from the tube may damage tissue if leg circulation is poor. A folded towel placed between the tube and skin can avoid this discomfort.

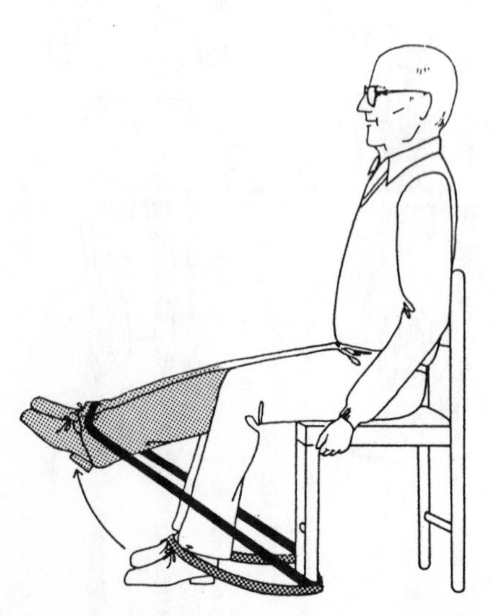

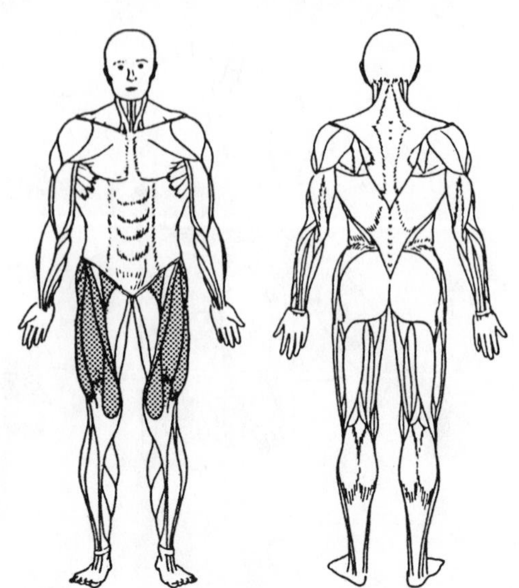

15. THE MULE KICK

7 8 10

Hook the inner tube under the back legs of your chair, as shown. This can't be done while sitting in the chair. Once the tube is in position stand behind your chair holding onto the back of the chair for support. Put one foot inside the loop and pull back away from the chair with your ankle. Feel the tube pressing on the back of your ankle. When the tube is stretched, return your leg toward the chair. Stretch the tube back five or six times, then step out of the inner tube. Place the other foot in the loop and repeat the exercise with your other leg. Since this exercise requires standing with your weight on one leg, it may be unsafe for you.

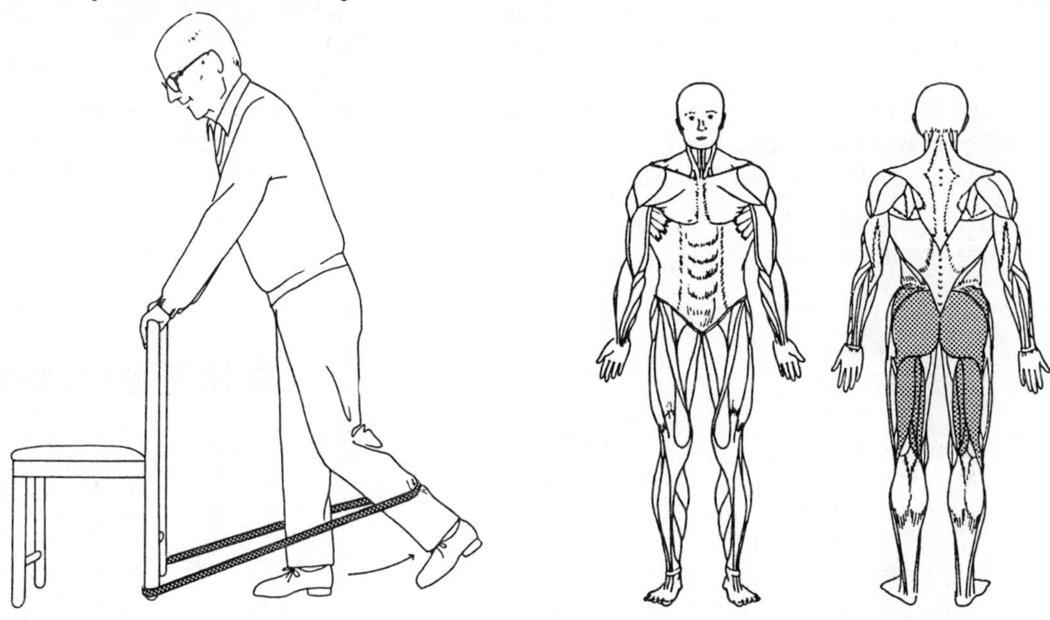

16. GRANDFATHER CLOCK

5 7 10

Hook the inner tube around the back legs of your chair as shown. Once the tube is in position stand behind your chair and use the back of the chair for support. Put one foot inside the loop and move that leg out to the side. Bring the leg back to the starting position and then repeat the pull sideways. Feel the tube pressing on the outside of your ankle. Keep your toes pointing forward or else you will not strengthen the intended muscles. Repeat this pull as many times as indicated in the activity plan then remove your foot from the tube. Place your other foot in the tube and pull outward as many times as directed. This exercise requires you to stand on one leg. That may be too hard for you, even though you are holding onto the chair. If it is unsafe for you, do not do the exercise. The "Spread your legs" exercise will strengthen the same muscles from a sitting position. Pressure from the tube may damage tissue if leg circulation is poor. A folded towel placed between the tube and skin can avoid this discomfort.

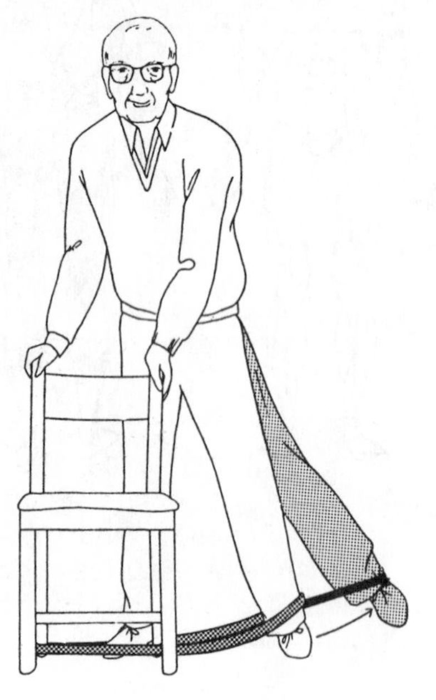

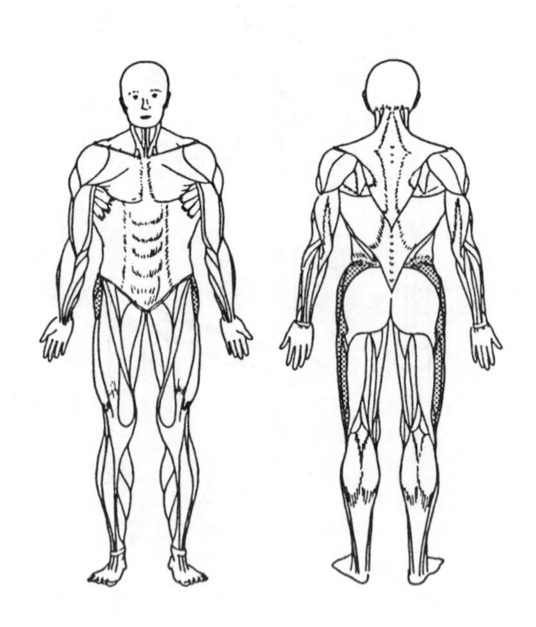

17. SPREAD YOUR LEGS

5 8 9 10

While sitting in your chair, put both feet inside the inner tube loop. Keep hold of the tube with your hands. Stretch your legs straight out in front of you on the floor. From this starting position spread your legs apart. As the tube stretches, feel it pressing on the outsides of your ankles. Once the tube is stretched, bring your legs together slowly.

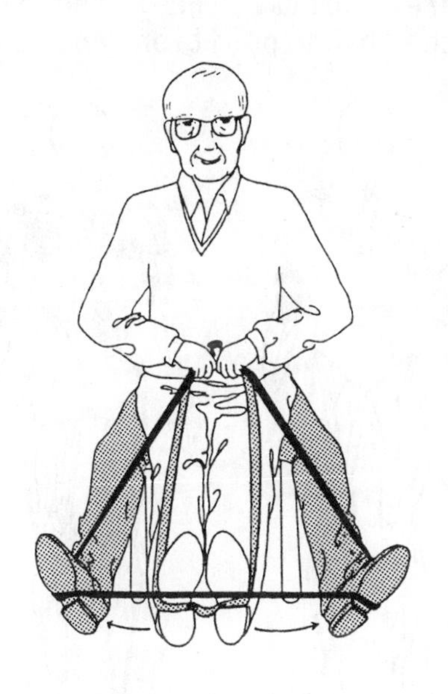

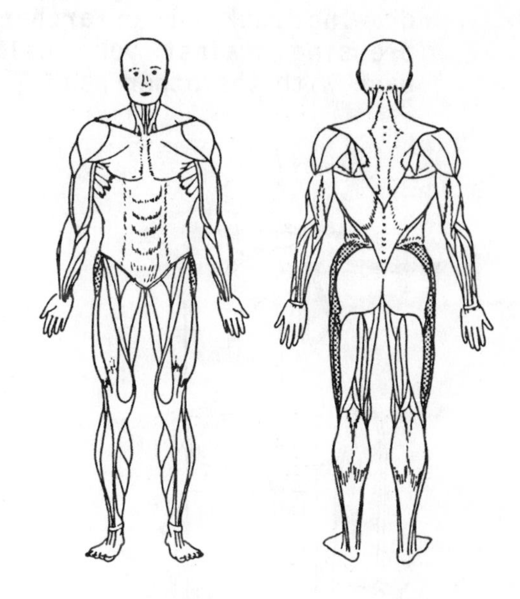

18. BRAKE YOUR CAR

5 7 10

While sitting in your chair, hold the tube in your hands like a horse's reins. Let the free loop of the tube rest on the floor and slip your toes only into the loop. Now stretch your legs out in front of you with the tube stretched under your toes as shown in the exercise illustration. Now move your feet forward to point your toes. Feel the tube pressing on the balls of your feet. Allow your toes to return slowly to point toward the ceiling. Repeat this pumping action.

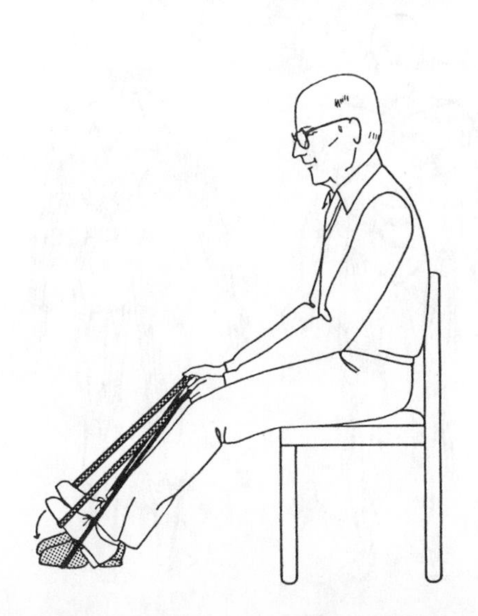

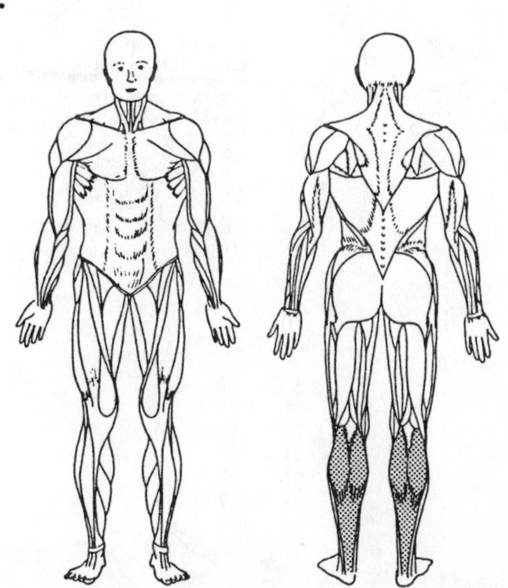

19. SHOOT THE ARROW

5 7

While sitting in a chair, place one hand inside the inner tube loop. Turn your palm away from you and stretch that arm out in front of you. With your free hand grasp both sides of the tube about halfway up the tube. See the exercise illustration for correct hand position. Keeping your arm straight in front of you, palm facing away, pull with the other arm as if you were drawing back on an archery bow for three pulls. Feel the tube pressing against your palm. Reverse the hand position and pull back with the other hand.

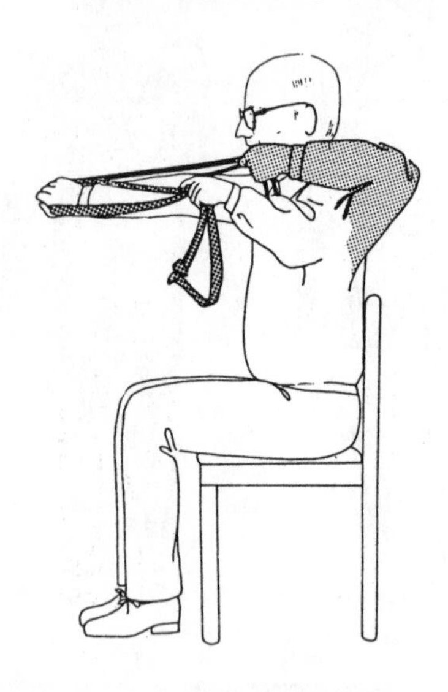

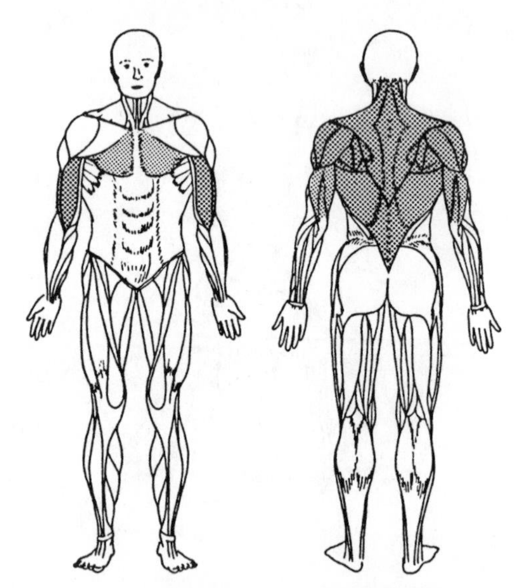

20. PULL ON YOUR SWEATER

5 7 9 10

While sitting in a chair, put both hands inside the loop formed by the tube, with the palms facing out. Raise your arms overhead and press outward, allowing the tube to stretch and pass behind your head. Return your arms overhead and press out again. As the arms move apart in this exercise, the elbows are allowed to bend.

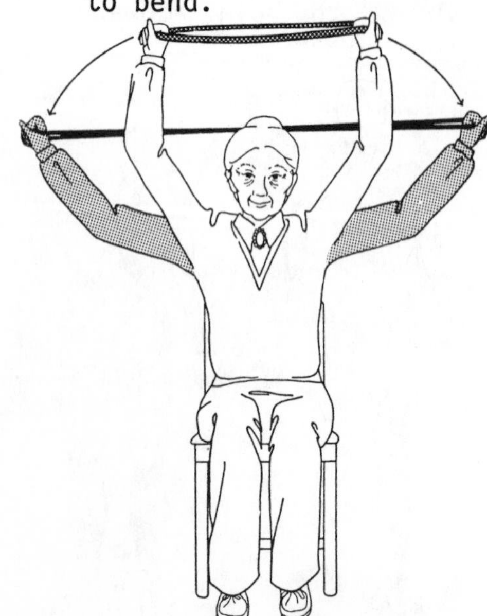

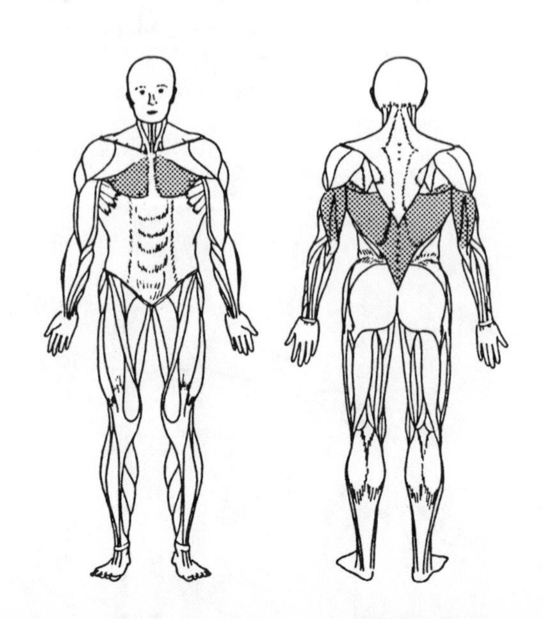

21. ROW-ROW-ROW YOUR BOAT

5 7 9

While sitting in your chair, hold the tube in your hands like a horse's reins. Let the free loop of the tube rest on the floor and slip your toes only into the loop. Now stretch your legs out in front of you with the tube stretched under your toes as shown in the exercise illustration. Pull your hands toward your chest, allowing your elbows to go out to the side. Straighten your arms and repeat.

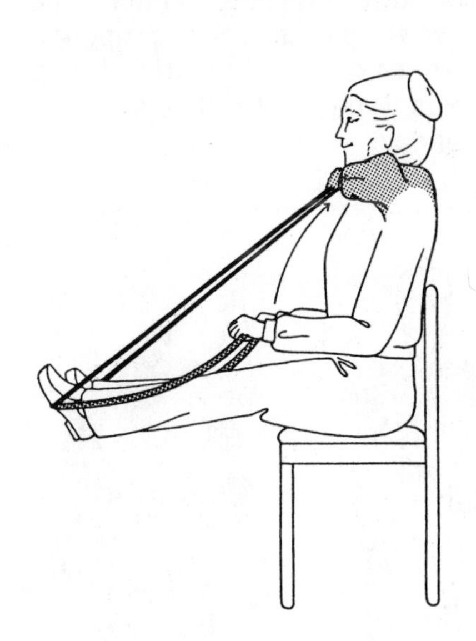

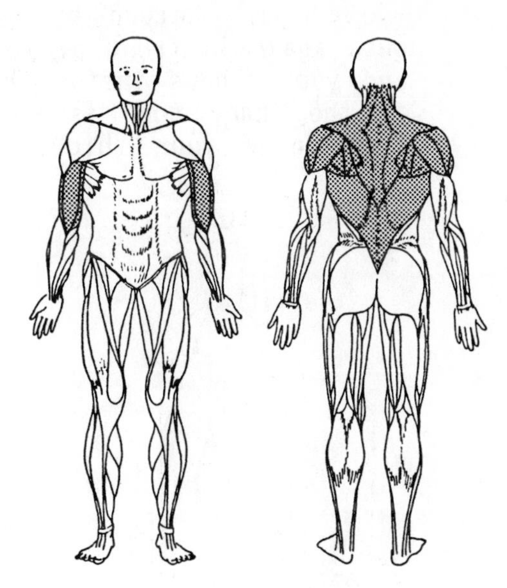

22. STRETCH AND YAWN

5 7 9

While sitting in your chair, slip both feet into the inner tube loop and work the tube up your legs until you have it around your upper thighs. Pull up on the tube, allowing your elbows to go inside the loop and your wrists to tip back pointing your palms toward the ceiling. This is the starting position for the exercise, which is diagrammed for you in the exercise illustration. From this position press the tube upward over your head. Return by bending your arms until your hands are once again in front of your chest. Keep your palms facing upward and your elbows inside the loop. This exercise is too difficult if the inner tube is short. The tube must be able to stretch from under your thighs to over your head.

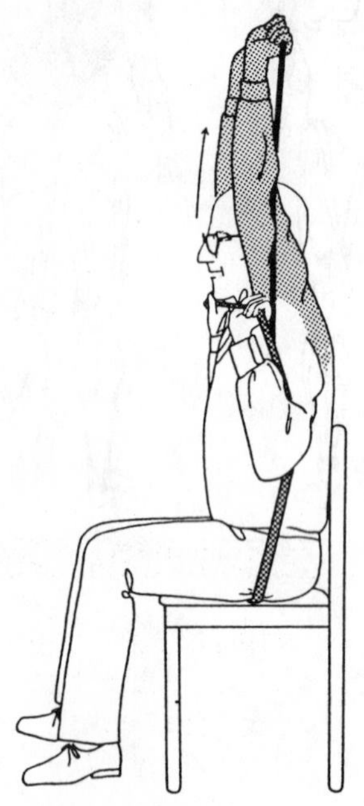

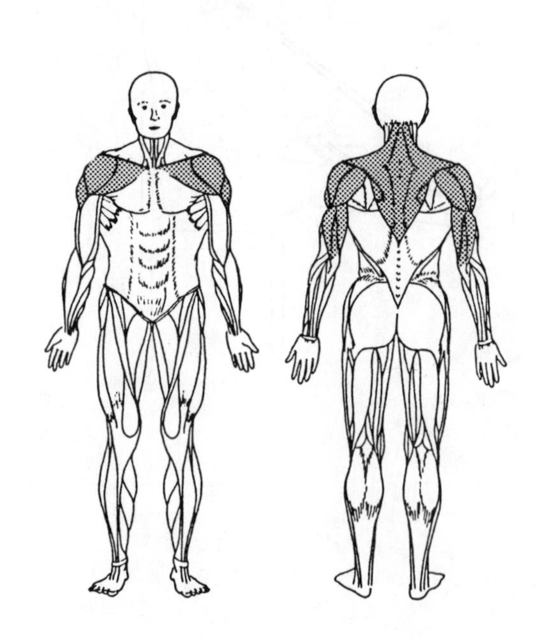

23. LIFT THE BARBELL

5 7 9

While sitting in a chair, hold the tube in your hands with your palms facing upward and the tube dangling in front of you. Step into the bottom of the tube loop with one or both feet. Bend your arms at the elbow and bring the tube toward your chin; then return your hands to your lap. Repeat this elbow bend, as weightlifters do when they perform the bicep curl exercise. Do you feel athletic? You are getting stronger!

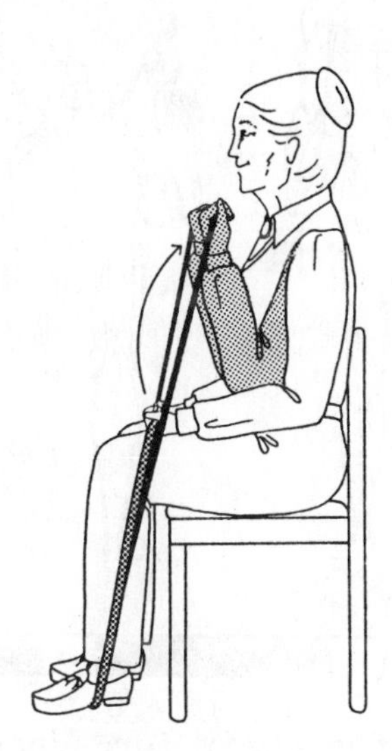

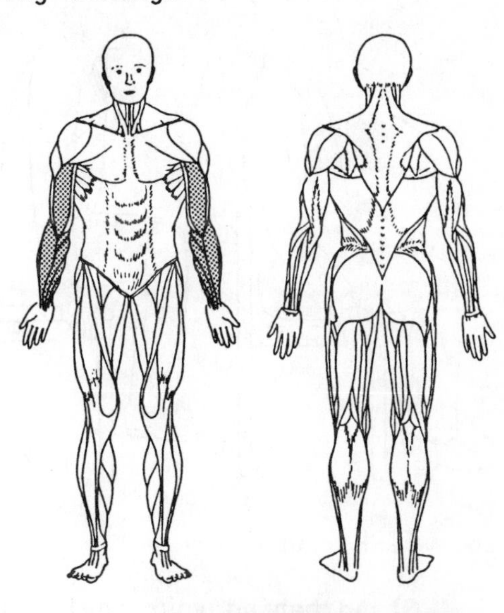

24. PLIÉ A LITTLE

3 8 10

Stand behind your chair, using the back of the chair for support. Point your toes outward as shown in the exercise illustration. From this position bend your knees slightly, directing your knees over your toes. Do not bend deep as the benefits from this exercise occur with only a minor dip. Return to a stand and repeat these dips .

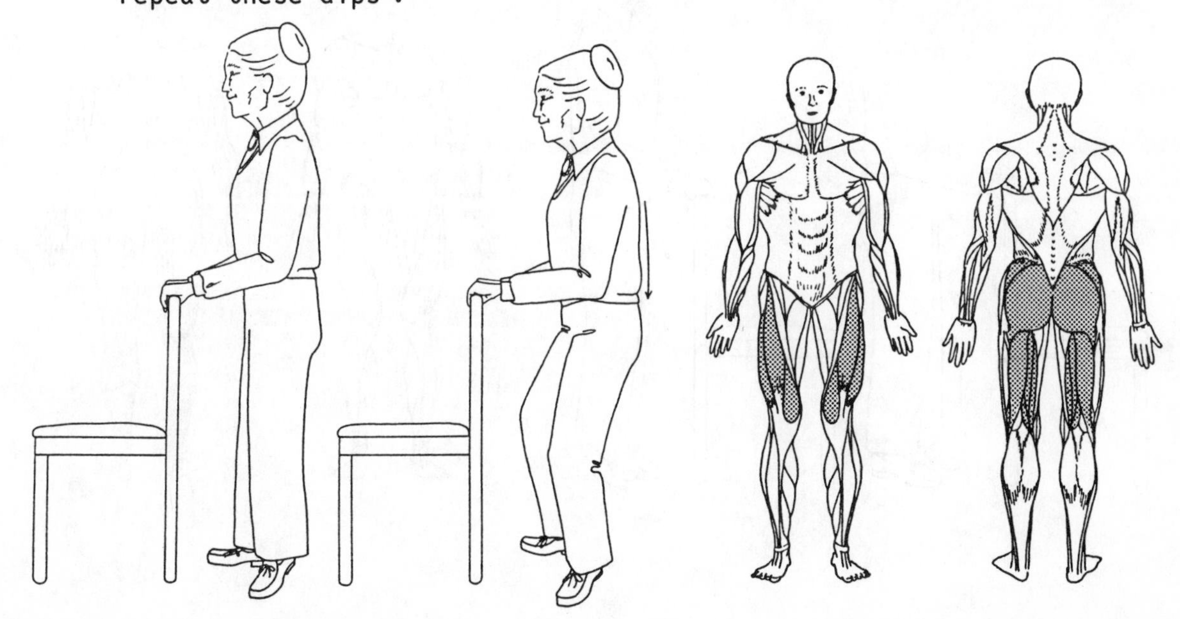

25. HOT SEAT

While seated in a chair grip firmly the sides of the chair seat. Press down on your arms and raise your buttocks off the chair seat. Lift only an inch or two and do the work with your arms. Lower back into the chair and repeat this lift.

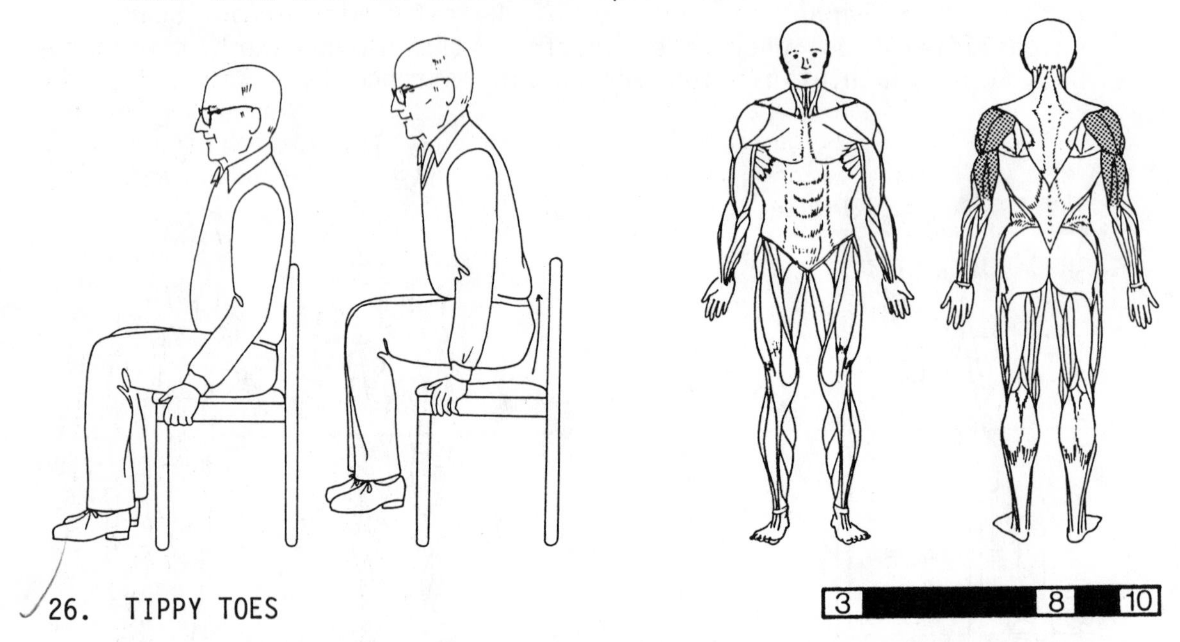

26. TIPPY TOES

3 8 10

Stand behind your chair and hold the back of the chair for support. Rise up on your toes slowly and lower back to the floor. Repeat this lift. If you feel unsafe even with the support of the chair, don't do this exercise. The same muscles can be strengthened with the "Brake your car" exercise.

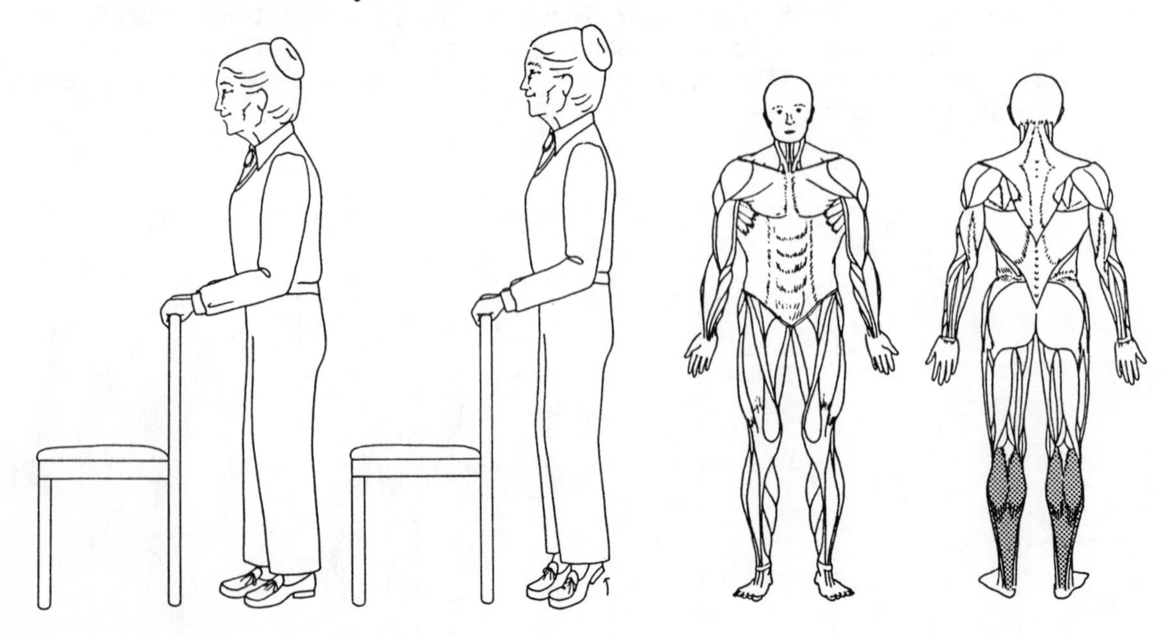

27. TIGHTEN YOUR TUMMY

4 8 10

From a seated position slide forward in your chair so that your buttocks are near the front edge of the seat and your upper back is leaning against the chair back. This is the slouching sitting posture your mother scolded you for using years ago! Hold onto the sides of the chair seat while you tuck your legs up off the floor. Raise your tucked legs slightly, then straighten them out in front. Now slowly lower your legs to the floor and begin another tuck. Do several of these if possible. Should the weight of both your legs be too much, try tucking, lifting, straightening, and lowering only one leg at a time. This is a strenuous exercise and requires a brief rest between lifts.

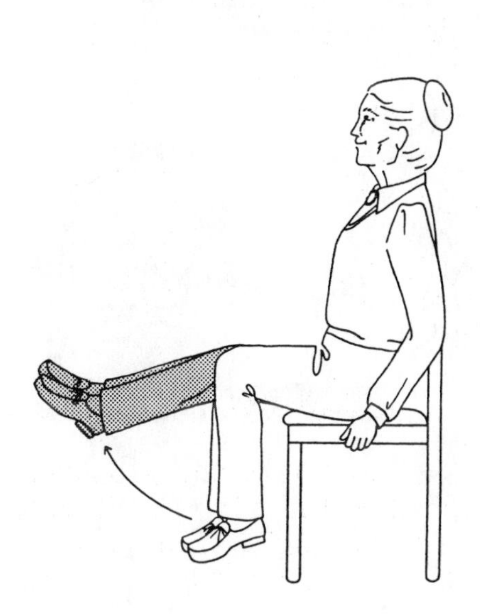

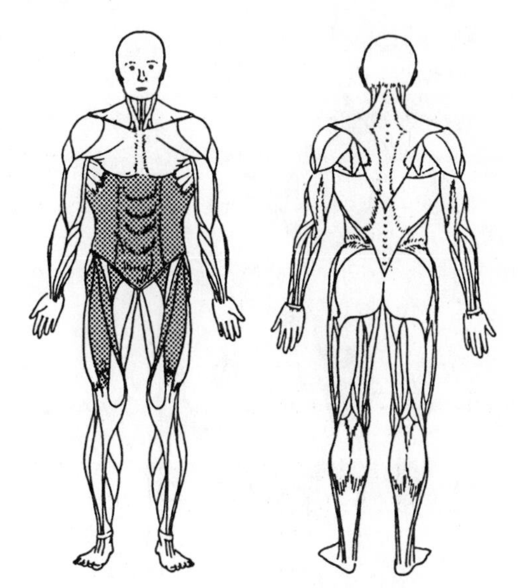

28. STAND UP AND SHOUT

Rise from a seated position to a stand several times. Try to avoid using your arms to help push up. If you must use your arms, try to make your legs do most of the work. This can be made easier by starting with your feet back under the chair, your buttocks scooted forward on the seat, your trunk leaning forward, and your arms stretched out in front as shown in the exercise illustration. If you are unstable when rising from this position, have the leader stand in front of you and guide your hands. When sitting down, always use your arms on the chair seat so that you don't fall back into the chair.

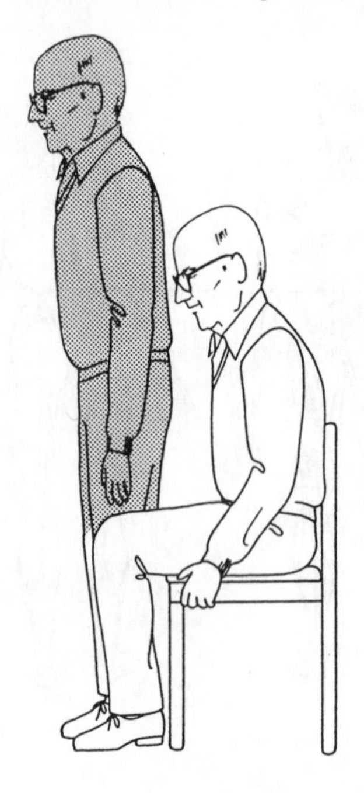

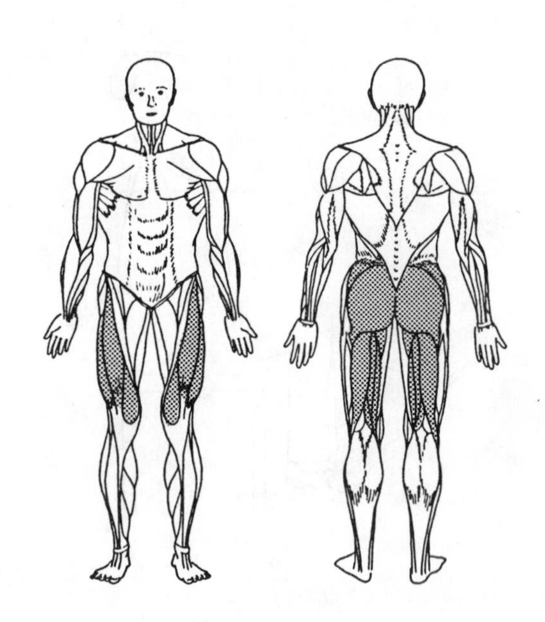

EXERCISE RECORD CHART

Exercise	3 re-peats	Extra work-out	5 re-peats	Extra work-out	6 re-peats	Extra work-out
1. Toast your arms						
2. Take a little drink						
3. Swing a garden gate						
4. Sitting jacks						
5. Swim the breast stroke						
6. Climb a rope						
7. Take off your hat						
8. Balance on a tightrope						
9. March a mile						
10. Kick the football						
11. Raise your toes						
12. Scissor your legs						
13. Flutter kick						
14. The bear trap						
15. The mule kick						
16. Grandfather clock						
17. Spread your legs						
18. Brake your car						
19. Shoot the arrow						
20. Pull on your sweater						
21. Row-row-row your boat						
22. Stretch and yawn						
23. Lift the barbell						
24. Plié a little						
25. Hot seat						
26. Tippy toes						
27. Tighten your tummy						
28. Stand up and shout						

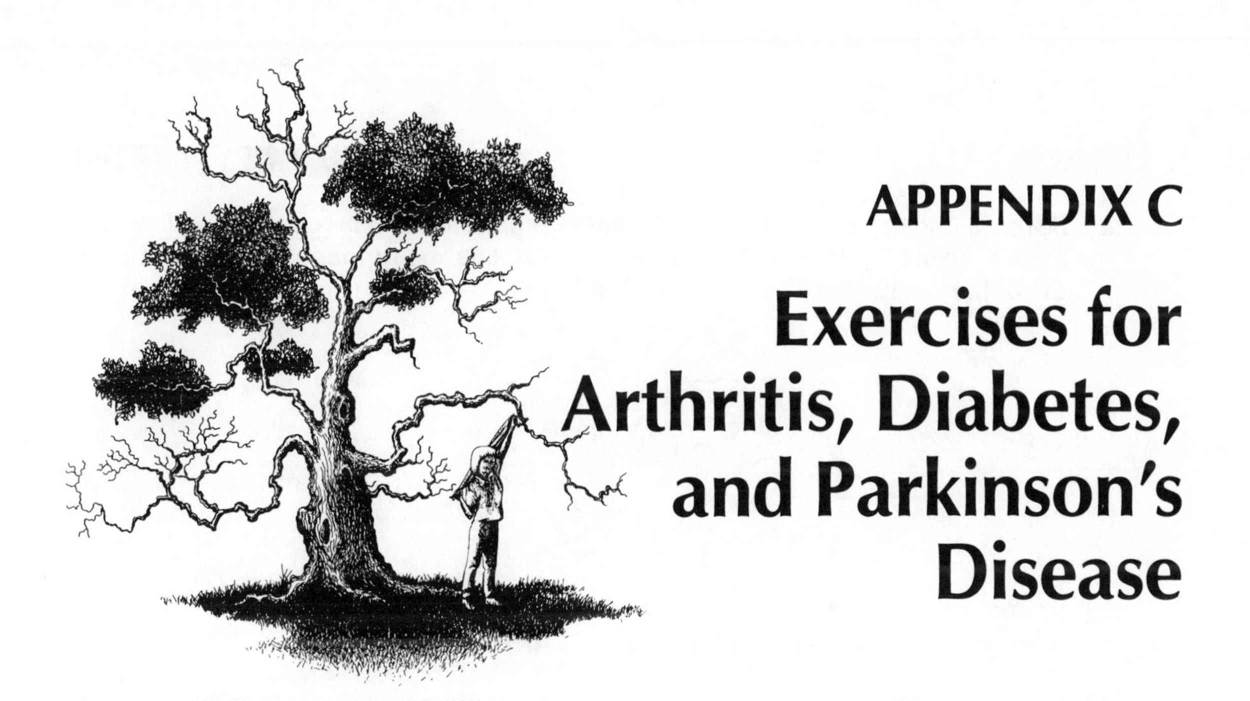

APPENDIX C

Exercises for Arthritis, Diabetes, and Parkinson's Disease

This appendix contains a description of each exercise and some illustrations. The bar code following the name of each exercise indicates for which activity plan that exercise is used. For example, if an exercise is used in ACTIVITY PLANS 4, 5, 6, 7, 8, 9, 10, then all boxes except 4 through 10 are darkened, as illustrated.

■	4	5	6	7	8	9	10

As the sessions progress, more and more exercises are added. Do only those that are approved by the physician. If all are approved, try to do as many as possible. There will be days when it is not possible to do some of the exercises due to pain or other illness. At these times it is best to rest until another time.

1. HANDS

7 8 9 10

(a) Hold a bean bag in each hand and knead it gently. For an added treat: in cold weather, warm the bean bags on a radiator or other warm spot before using them.

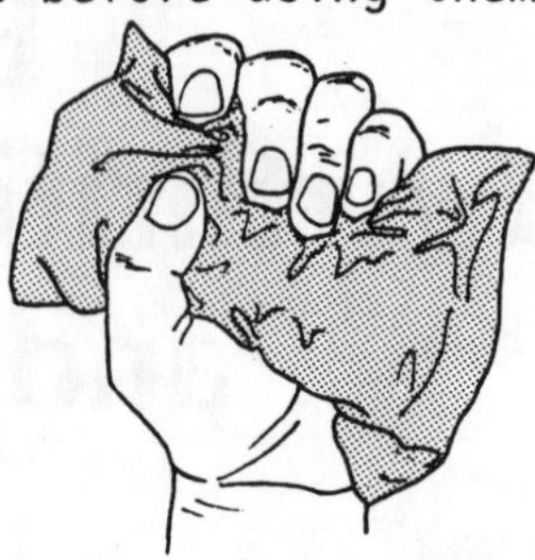

(b) Drumming your fingers. Put your fingers through the motions of playing the piano or using a typewriter.

(c) Like a fan opening and closing, spread your fingers apart and then bring them back together.

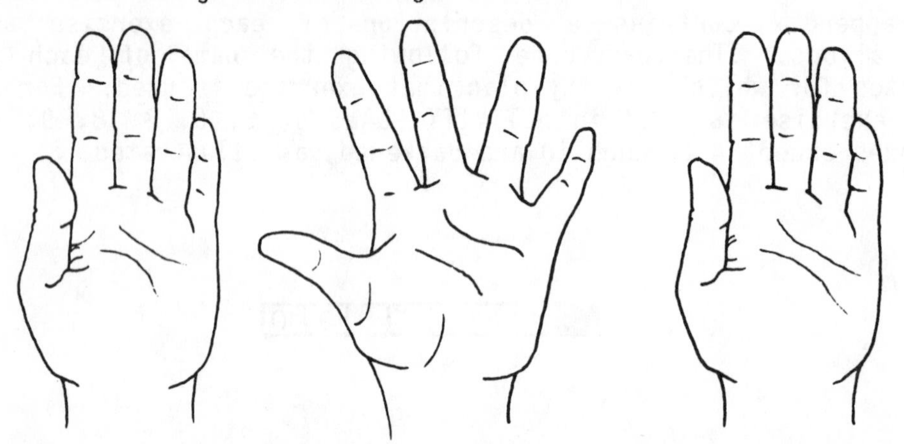

(d) Gently press the tip of each finger against the thumb. Go back and forth from index finger, to middle finger, to ring finger, to pinky finger.

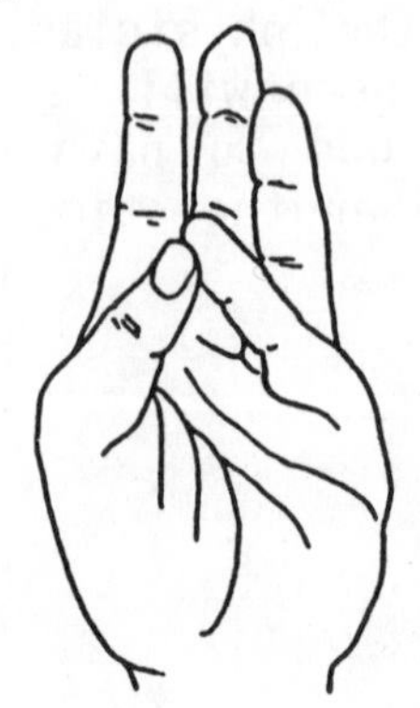

(e) With each finger make tiny circles clockwise and counterclockwise. This takes real concentration! Don't skip any fingers!

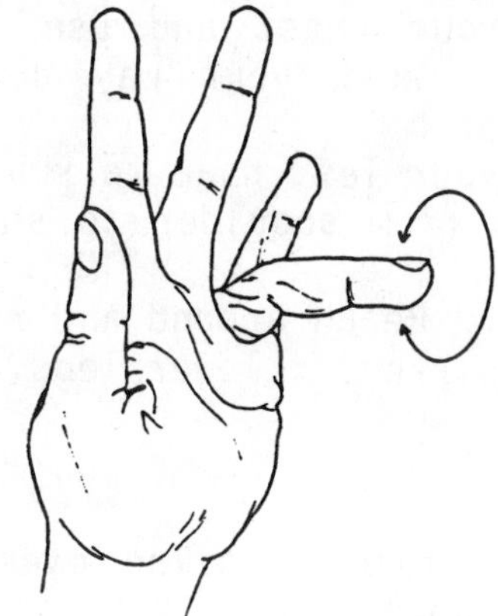

(f) Making circles from the wrist. Draw an imaginary circle with each hand, make the movement as round and full as possible.

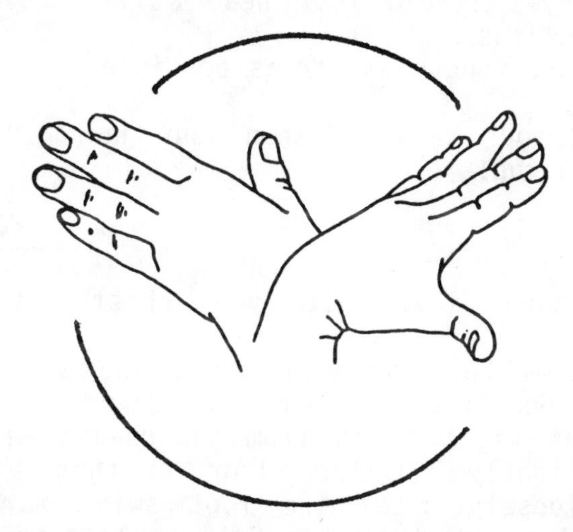

(g) Lightly rub the palms and back of your hands as though applying hand lotion.

(h) Lightly flick your hands as though flicking water off.

2. MASSAGE | 3 | 4 | 5 | 6 | 7 | 8 | 9 | 10 |

Using the gentle kneading and drumming action of your fingers, this will "wake up" your entire body. Take it slowly. Pay attention to the area being massaged; notice whether it is tight or sore. Try to mentally relax the tight muscles as you massage them. Pay particular attention to joints; cup your hands and gently rub in circles over the knees, elbows, shoulders, wrists, and ankles.

(a) Begin with a scalp rub. Be sure to do your entire head.
(b) Lightly rub your face. Don't overlook your jaws, temples, and forehead.

(c) Yes, rub your ears too!
(d) Gently rub the back of your neck up into the hairline. Do not rub directly on bones but around them.
(e) Reach across your chest and use your right hand to rub your left shoulder. Work your way down your arm to your elbow, wrist, and hand.
(f) Repeat, using your left hand to rub your right.
(g) Rub your chest from shoulder to shoulder and down the midpoint (sternum).
(h) Rub your sides. Reach around and rub your lower back.
(i) Rub your thighs, knees, lower legs, ankles, and feet.

3. FACE

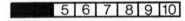

(a) Pucker up your face, closing eyes tightly; then stretch eyes and mouth wide open.
(b) Move your mouth from side to side and up and down.
(c) Raise and lower your eyebrows.
(d) Move your eyes. Hold your head still as you move your eyes in all directions.
(e) Stick out your tongue as far as possible.
(f) Wink!
(g) Lightly rub your temples, then your jaws. Let your jaws hang loose as you rub.

4. RAG DOLL

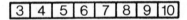

(a) Hold your hands level with your chest and let them go limp from the wrist.
(b) Let your arms hang by your sides and swing freely from the shoulders. Gently swing them forward and backward a few times.
(c) Support your right thigh from underneath with both hands and lift it slightly off the floor so that the foot and lower leg hang loosely. Let the foot swing forward and backward and in circles. Do the same with the left thigh.
(d) Let your head, shoulders, and arms hang forward slightly as your chin rests on your chest. Swing your arms gently.
(e) S-L-O-W-L-Y straighten back up, lift your head, and assume an erect posture.

5. NECK 4 5 6 7 8 9 10

(a) Sit comfortably, hands in lap, posture erect but not tense, and keep your body still as you move your head through this series of exercises.

(b) "Yes"--S-L-O-W-L-Y lift your chin up slightly toward the ceiling and back down toward your chest. Repeat.

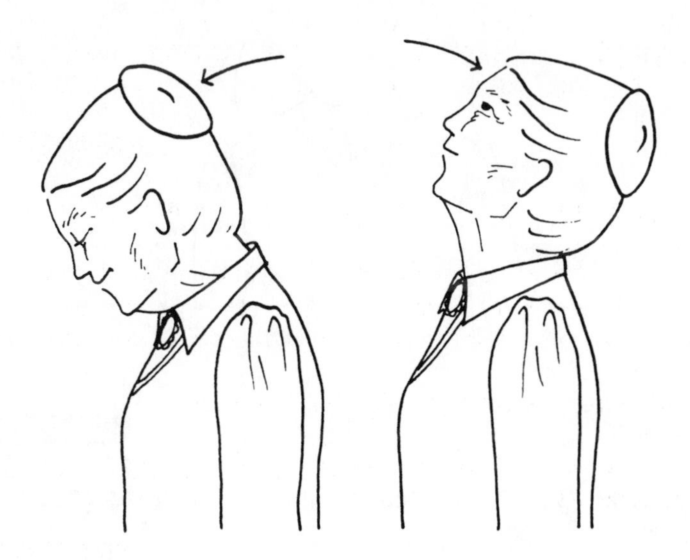

(c) "No"--S-L-O-W-L-Y move your chin over to one shoulder and then to the other shoulder. Repeat.

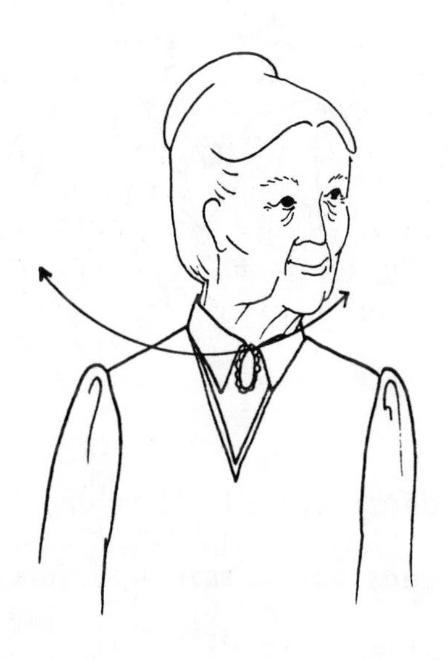

(d) "Maybe"--S-L-O-W-L-Y drop your right ear toward the right shoulder and then your left ear toward the left shoulder. Try to keep your shoulders down while doing this. Repeat.

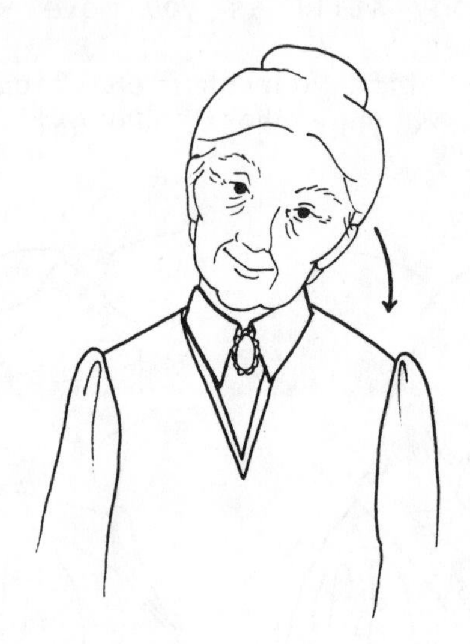

6. SHOULDER SHRUGS

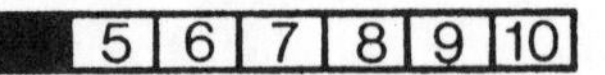

S-L-O-W-L-Y lift your shoulders up as high as possible and lower them back down. Repeat.

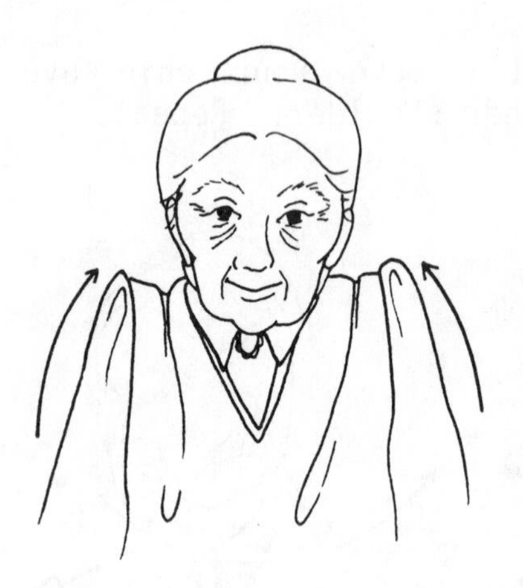

7. SHOULDER ROLLS

4 5 6 7 8 9 10

(a) Move your shoulders forward, then up, back and down to starting position.
(b) Move your shoulders back, then up, forward and down to starting position.
(c) Repeat in both directions.

8. GOOD MORNING STRETCH | 5 | 6 | 7 | 8 | 9 | 10 |

(a) Using S-L-O-W, continuous motion, breathe deeply and enjoy this stretch thoroughly:
(b) From your sides, lift your arms forward, up to shoulder level then overhead as you inhale. Exhale as you move your arms S-L-O-W-L-Y out to the sides and down to starting position. Repeat.

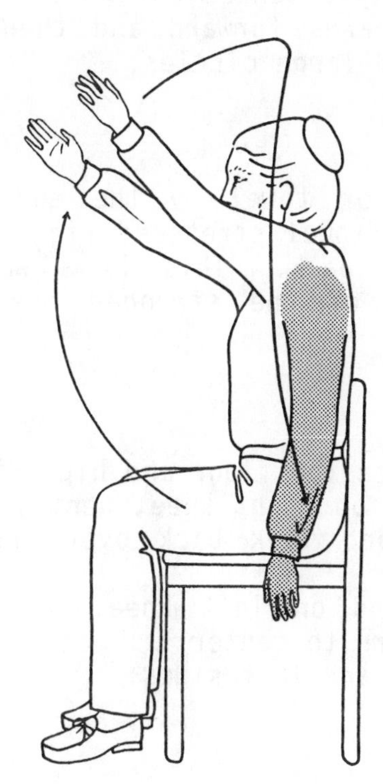

9. PALMS UP, PALMS DOWN | 7 | 8 | 9 | 10 |

With arms extended forward at shoulder level, rotate palms up to face the ceiling and down to face the floor.

10. ELBOW BENDS | 7 | 8 | 9 | 10 |

With arms extended straight forward at shoulder level, palms up, bring your fingers up to touch your shoulders, then straighten your elbows and move hands back out to starting position. Repeat.

11. ELBOW TOUCHES | 7 | 8 | 9 | 10 |

Begin with fingers resting on your shoulders, elbows lifted up and pointed forward, parallel to each other. Move elbows apart and out to the sides, reaching back as far as possible, then bring elbows to the front and try to touch them lightly together. Repeat.

12. ELBOW CIRCLES 7 8 9 10

Begin with fingers resting on your shoulders, elbows out to the sides. S-L-O-W-L-Y circle your elbows forward and then backward.

13. ARM CIRCLES 7 8 9 10

Begin with arms fully extended out to the sides at shoulder level. S-L-O-W-L-Y circle arms forward and then backward. Do a series of small circles and large circles.

14. SCARF/TOWEL 7 8 9 10

Holding the scarf or towel by the ends or corners, move arms up and down keeping towel stretched tight. Reach back and "towel" your shoulders and back. This is a way of exercising a weak arm with the help of the stronger one. When finished, shake out both arms.

15. TORSO TWIST 4 5 6 7 8 9 10

(a) Keep feet flat on the floor and hips firmly on the chair.
(b) Place left hand on right knee, gently twist head and shoulders to the right and look back over the right shoulder. Then return to center.
(c) Place right hand on left knee and look back over the left shoulder. Return to center.
(d) Repeat to right and left sides.

16. SIDE STRETCHES 5 6 7 8 9 10

(a) Sit erect with your feet on the floor in front of you, arms hanging by your sides.
(b) Drop your head to your right shoulder, then drop your shoulder and head down a little lower, going only as far as you comfortably can. Try not to lean forward as you bend sideward.
(c) S-L-O-W-L-Y straighten up to the starting position.
(d) Repeat to the other side.
(e) To modify: Bring left arm up as you bend to the left, right arm up as you bend to the right.

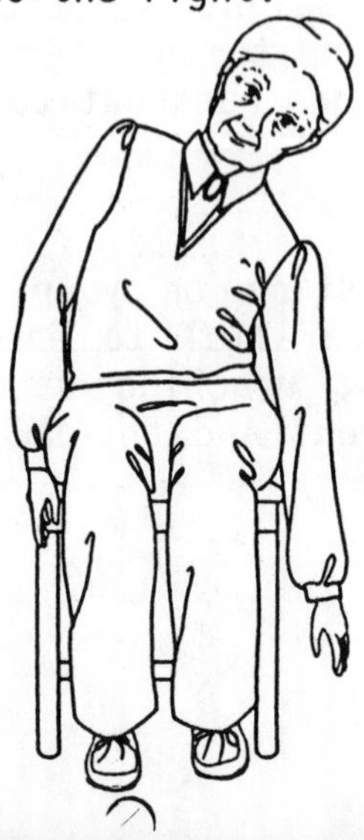

17. LEGS

4 5 6 7 8 9 10

NOT RECOMMENDED FOR THOSE WITH HIP REPLACEMENT

(a) With both hands supporting the right thigh from below, pull it up toward the chest as far as possible; then lower it back to the chair.
(b) Place hands under the left thigh, pull it up toward the chest as far as possible; then lower it back to the chair.
(c) Repeat right and left sides.

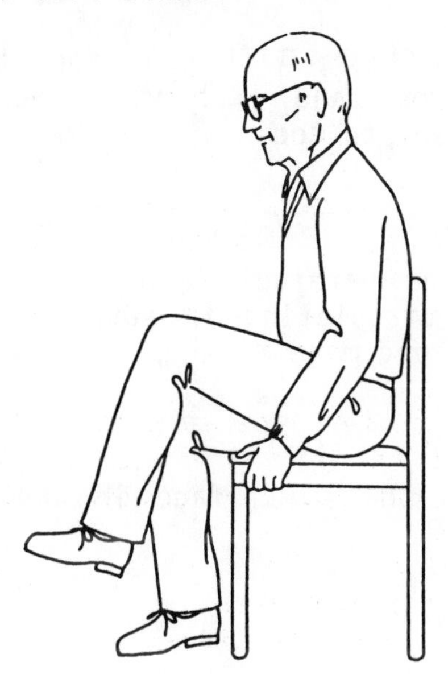

18. WALK IN PLACE

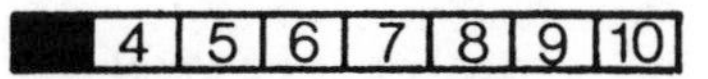

Sit comfortably erect, hold the sides of the chair and lift one knee and then the other for 8 counts, with each knee lift receiving 1 count. Move S-L-O-W-L-Y and only within comfortable range.

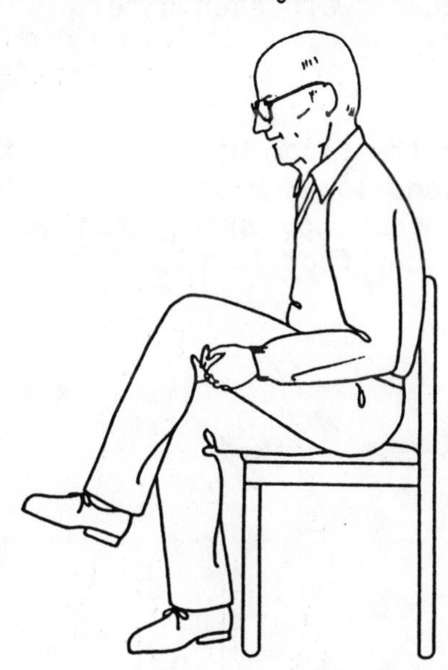

19. ANKLE ROTATIONS 4 5 6 7 8 9 10

(a) Raise your right foot up off the floor and move it in circles, clockwise and then counterclockwise.
(b) Raise your left foot up off the floor and move it in circles, clockwise and counterclockwise. Move the foot as far in all directions as possible. Imagine drawing circles with your toes.

20. HEEL AND TOE LIFTS 6 7 8 9 10

With heels on the floor, lift your toes up as high as possible; then lower your toes and lift your heels. Go back and forth a few times from heel to toe.

21. TOE WIGGLES 6 7 8 9 10

These are best done barefooted, but can be done with shoes on, to get the blood circulating in your toes! Just move your toes as far as possible and move them up and down.

22. FOOT CURLS 6 7 8 9 10

Move your feet so the soles face in and out. Alternate in and out several times.

23. INCHWORM 6 7 8 9 10

Inch your feet forward by curling and uncurling your toes.

24. THE CHARLESTON 6 7 8 9 10

Begin with feet together. Use the rocking motion of the heel-to-toe exercise, move heels and toes sideways away from each other, then back toward each other.

25. LEG LIFTS--FORWARD 9 10

(a) Begin seated on the floor with your feet in front of you.
(b) Lift your knee and lower your foot to the floor. Repeat.
(c) Lift your left foot up, straighten your knee, then bend your knee and lower your foot to the floor. Repeat.

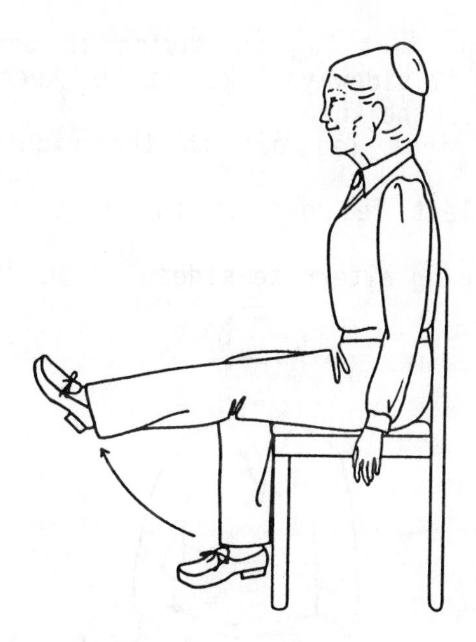

(d) Extend both feet forward and up, straighten your knees, and then bend your knees and lower your feet to the floor.

26. SINGLE LEG REACHES TO THE SIDE

(a) Begin seated with your feet on the floor in front of you.
(b) Straighten your right leg and reach out to the right side with it; then bring it back to the front and lower your foot. Repeat.
(c) Reach forward and out to the left side with your left leg in the same way; then bring it back to the front and lower your foot. Repeat.

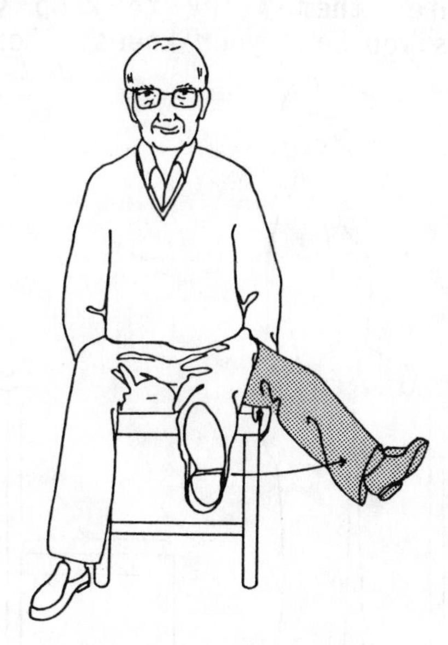

27. HIP JOINT

9 10

(a) Think of your bent leg as moving in one piece from the hip joint; swing it sideways like a gate, keeping your foot hanging directly under the knee.
(b) Swing your right leg out to the right side and then back to the front.
(c) Swing your left leg out to the left side and then back to the front.
(d) Repeat, swinging alternate sides.

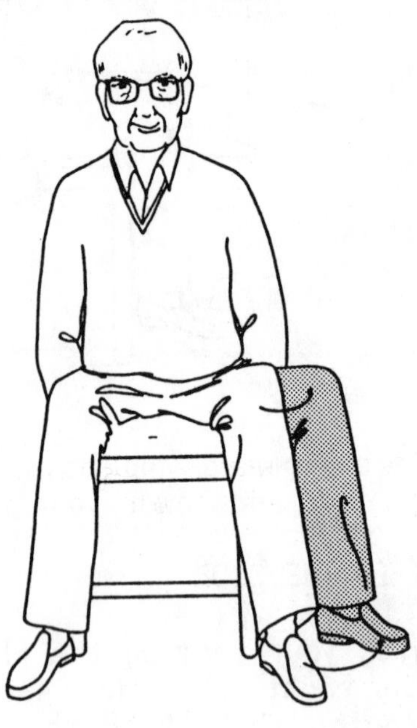

28. STANDING KNEE BENDS

9 10

(a) Stand beside or behind a chair.
(b) Keeping your heels on the floor, bend your knees slightly then straighten them. Try to keep your knees from touching each other as you bend your knees. Repeat.

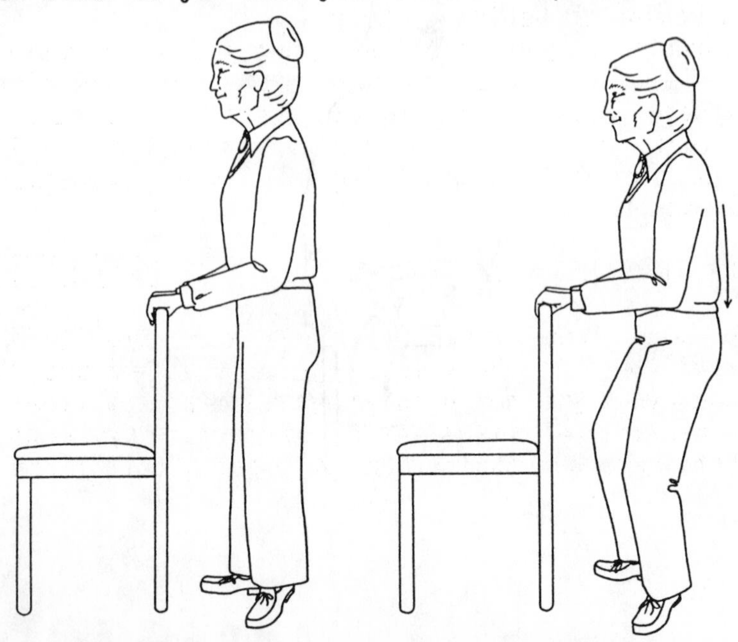

29. STANDING TOE RAISES 9 10

(a) Stand beside or behind a chair.
(b) With your legs straight, roll up onto the balls of your feet; then gently lower your heels back to the floor.

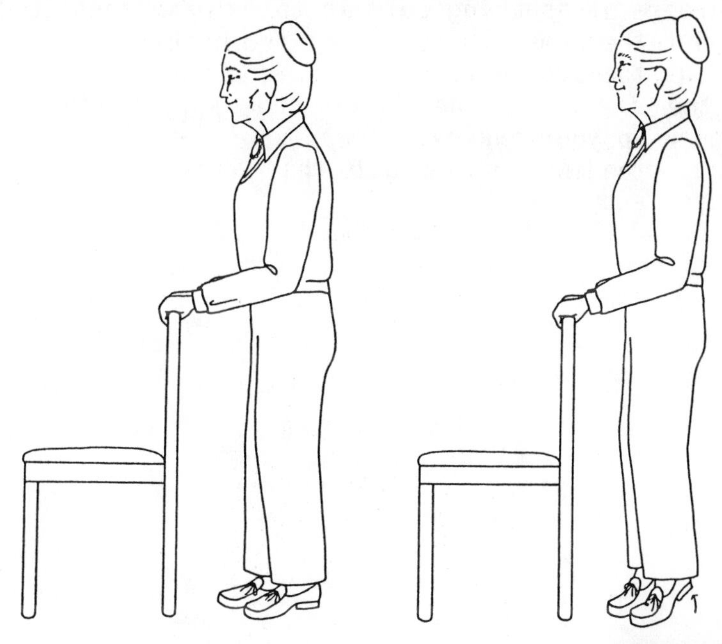

30. STANDING KNEE BEND/TOE RAISES 9 10

(a) Stand beside or behind a chair.
(b) Keep heels on the floor; bend knees slightly, then straighten them.
(c) Lift heels up and raise onto the balls of your feet; lower heels. Repeat.

31. HIP CIRCLES 9 10

(a) Stand beside or behind a chair.
(b) With hands on your hips and your knees slightly bent, move your hips in a wide circle. Move hips in circles to the right and then around to the left. Make sure it is your hips that are moving and not your shoulders! If you don't have a mirror to check with, ask your exercise partner to check you.

32. WHOLE BODY STRETCHES 3 4 5 6 7 8 9 10

(a) These are free-form, full-body stretches. There is no "correct" way to do this. The only rules are that it feel good and that you not hold your breath at any time!
(b) S-L-O-W-L-Y move and stretch one part of your body and then another; remember to include every part, both large and small.

(c) Move everything that can move; reach with it, stretch it as far as is comfortable.

33. SHAKE OUT

(a) The purpose of "shaking out" is to release tension.
(b) Shake out the arms, loosen up at the joints.
(c) Shake out the shoulders.
(d) Lift the feet off the floor and gently flutter them, try to loosen up your ankles.
(e) If done standing, shake out the limbs as above but include the torso and hips.

FLORIDA STATE UNIVERSITY
3 1254 00761 0534

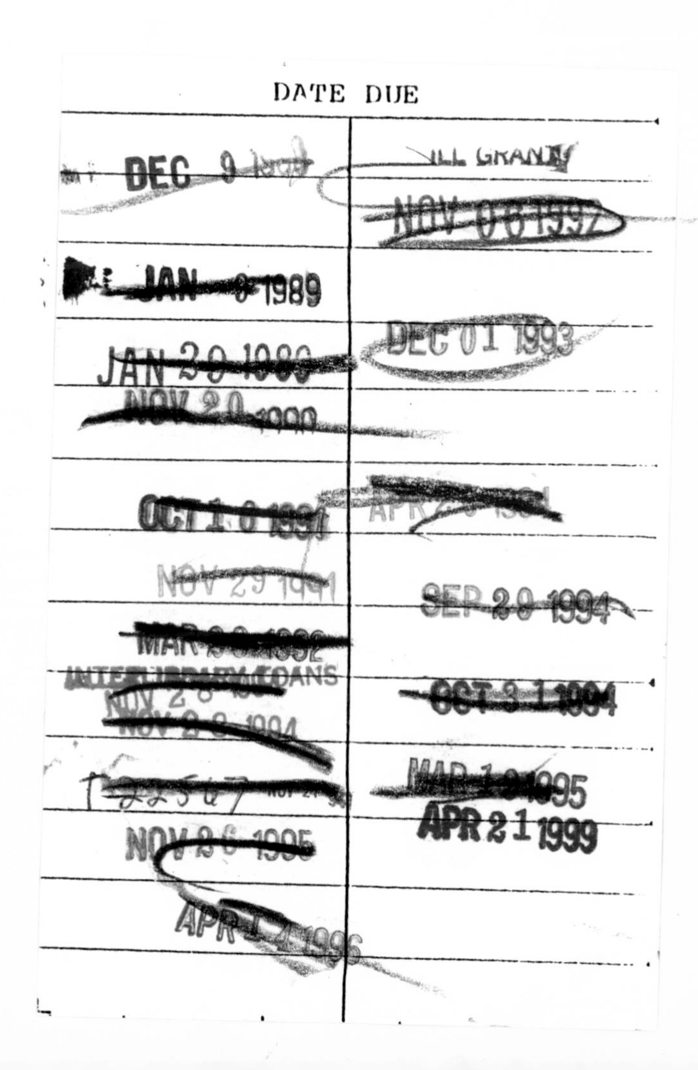
DATE DUE

Volume Nineteen in the Springer Series on

ADULTHOOD AND AGING

EXERCISE ACTIVITIES for the ELDERLY

Kay Flatten, P.E.D., **Barbara Wilhite,** Ed.D., **Eleanor Reyes-Watson,** M.A.

Here is a handy resource for those working directly with institutionalized and homebound elders. A variety of exercises are presented, some of which are geared to clients with such conditions as arthritis, diabetes, and Parkinson's disease, and others which are designed to build up muscular strength and maintain flexibility. Included are guidelines for conducting an exercise program, information on community resource referral, illustrations, exercise charts, and activity plans.

Of related interest from Springer

RECREATION ACTIVITIES for the ELDERLY

Kay Flatten, P.E.D., **Barbara Wilhite,** Ed.D., **Eleanor Reyes-Watson,** M.A.

This easy-to-follow guide presents a wide range of recreational activities appropriate for homebound and institutionalized elders. Included in this volume are simple crafts that utilize easily obtainable, inexpensive materials; hobbies focusing on collections, nature, and the arts; and games emphasizing both mental and physical activity. The activity plans include: block printing, guessing games, indoor golf, astronomy, music appreciation, letter writing, reading aloud, remembering the past, poetry, and much more.

Communication Skills for Working with Elders

Barbara Bender Dreher, Ph.D.

This book provides a practical guide to effective interaction with the elderly and presents techniques for overcoming common communication problems and disorders found among aging persons. Emphasizing skills development, the author explores the physical, social, and emotional changes that can create unique communication needs. Written in a clear and readable style, this book is excellent for source use in departments of gerontology, social work, nursing, and communication.

A Basic Guide to Working with Elders

Michael J. Salamon, Ph.D.

Designed as an introductory guide for gerontological service providers, this concise book helps answer practical questions on the mental health needs of the aged and social support systems. Readers learn how to assess community needs, how to intervene with older adults, and how to evaluate program effectiveness. Detailed suggestions are given on establishing recreation and socialization programs. Useful as a text for students or as a basic resource for the beginning field worker.

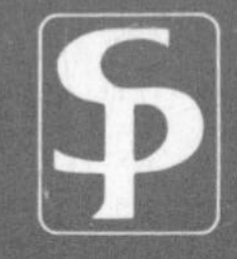

SPRINGER PUBLISHING COMPANY
536 Broadway, New York, NY 10012-3955 • (212) 431-4370

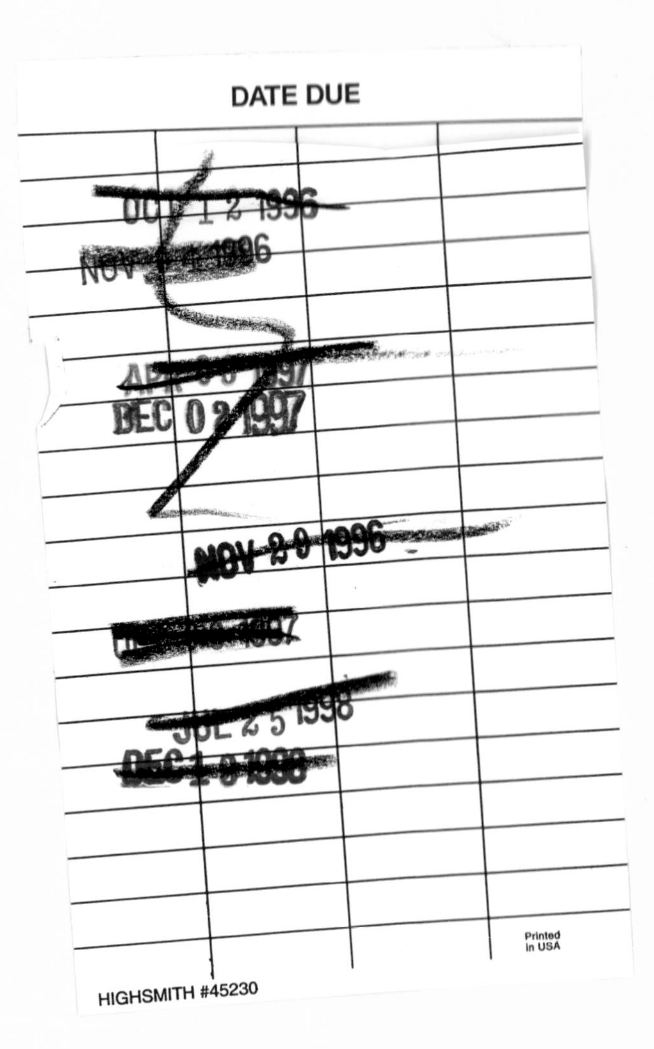